The Midwife and the Bereaved Family

The Midwife and the Bereaved Family

Jane Warland

Ausmed Publications
Melbourne

Australasian Health Education Systems Pty Ltd
(ACN 005 611 626)
trading as
Ausmed Publications
275–277 Mount Alexander Road
Ascot Vale, Victoria 3032, Australia

Further copies of this book and of all other Ausmed publications are
available from the Distribution Manager, Ausmed Publications,
PO Box 4086, Melbourne University, Parkville, Victoria 3052, Australia.
Telephone +613/(03) 9375 7311.
Fax +613/(03) 9375 7299.
E-mail ausmed@ausmed.com.au
Home page www.ausmed.com.au

NATIONAL LIBRARY OF AUSTRALIA

Cataloguing-in-Publication entry

Warland, Jane, 1957-.
The midwife and the bereaved family.

Includes index.
ISBN 0 9577988 0 6

1. Mothers - Counseling of. 2. Fathers – Counseling of. 3. Midwives. 4. Infants
(Newborn) – Death – Psychological aspects. 5. Pregnancy – Psychological
aspects. I. Title.

618.2

Edited by Robyn Whiteley and John Collins, The WC Company Pty Ltd
Cover, design, typesetting and printing by
Hyde Park Press, 4 Deacon Avenue, Richmond, South Australia 5033,
telephone (08) 8234 2044, fax (08) 8234 1887,
e-mail sales@hydeparkpress.com.au
Text set in 11/14 Garamond

FOREWORD

A dead baby is a very real happening for some women and midwives. This death may occur in early, middle or late pregnancy, at birth or in the postnatal period. Miscarriage, abortion and stillbirth are the terms used to describe this event in a woman's life. Technology and sophisticated prenatal care have helped to reduce infant morbidity and mortality in Australia. But however good the technology and care may be, when a woman and her family are faced with a dead baby they will ask many questions of both themselves and the caregivers; perhaps not immediately, but they will ask. What midwives need to ask of themselves is 'Do I have the knowledge, the skills and the ability to deal with questions?'

I can recall my first baby being born in Singapore at fifteen weeks' gestation. I experienced labour for seven hours and then a curette and eventual discharge from hospital. No family or close friends were there, just my husband, me and a nun who kept telling me to 'Stop crying, you are young enough to get pregnant again'. I put this experience out of my mind for many years and it resurfaced some five years ago when I was triggered to think how old that baby boy would have been now. I did not name him, as I didn't realise that I could, and I didn't dispose of his body, as I didn't know I could. I did see him and for that I am grateful. The lived experience of women who have birthed a dead baby is that they need support and care that is appropriate to the time and the situation. This book provides strategies for midwives to care for women like me to ensure a positive outcome of the birthing experience.

This book is based on women's experiences and has been written for midwives, by a midwife. The chapters follow a chronological pattern from early pregnancy loss through to late pregnancy loss. The chapter on subsequent pregnancy is useful as a guide for the midwife who will be caring for that woman and her family. Nothing is overlooked in this book as the appendices give helpful hints and strategies for looking after yourself, men partners, children and grandparents. So often these groups are forgotten in texts and the focus is always on the woman. The cultural section provides an overview of some of the mores and rules of particular cultural and religious groups and will be very helpful to guide care in a sensitive way.

The inclusion of research articles and recommended reading will give midwives the opportunity to read in more depth areas that appeal and are prominent in their practice. The checklists provide an easy reference to ensure best practice while maintaining an empathy for the woman and her family. There are some arguable points in the text that will challenge midwives' thinking and practice.

This book is an extension of the work already begun by Jane and builds on her first two books *Pregnancy After Loss* and *Our Baby Died*. Jane is to be congratulated for putting her thoughts, the experiences of others, and research together to produce a book that is easy to read and full of hints to care for the woman and her family who birth a dead baby. Contributing to the literature on this difficult topic is commendable.

Pauline Glover

Pauline Glover
Registered Nurse, Registered Midwife, Diploma of Teaching (Nurse Education), Bachelor of Education, Master of Nursing Science, Doctor of Education (submitted for examination), Fellow of the Australian College of Midwives
Senior Lecturer in Midwifery, Flinders University, Adelaide, South Australia, and Editor, *Australian College of Midwives Inc. Journal.*

PS I have two wonderful adult children and one grandchild, with another grandchild due in September, and I thank God for all this.

CONTENTS

APPENDIX 5 CULTURAL/RELIGIOUS CONSIDERATIONS 138

HANDY LISTS

ACKNOWLEDGEMENTS

There are a large number of people who have made contributions to this book. Some have told me their stories, others have read and commented on a chapter or section. I thank them all for generously sharing their thoughts and experiences with me.

I want to thank several people who have made a significant contribution to this book.

Our first baby, whom we call Lesley, is the inspiration behind the first chapter.

Several parents bereaved through genetic termination were kind enough to read the manuscript and make comments. I particularly would like to thank Susan Whitehead, a woman whom I have not met face to face, who was kind enough not only to read the chapter but also to share her story with me. This helped me understand some of the trials and tribulations of continuing a pregnancy after poor fetal prognosis.

Our baby Emma, who was stillborn at term, is not only the inspiration behind Chapter 3, but also the motivation for the entire book.

Karon Lloyd kindly gave me her permission to dissect her video *A part of you dies* to use from it some significant quotes.

My friend and fellow author Lynne Schulz was kind enough to read and make constructive comments on Chapter 4 as well as give her permission to use quotes from her book *The Diary*.

My pregnancy with Sarah, our subsequent child, gave me insight into the needs of bereaved families who are pregnant again after the death of a baby.

I have re-used much material from *Pregnancy after Loss*, the book that I wrote with my husband and self-published in 1996. I wish to thank all the families who contributed to that book and who were happy for their quotes to be used in this book.

Wherever you find quotes in italics throughout this book, they will usually be quotes from mothers or families whose babies have died. Quotes from other sources (books, conference papers etc.) are in the same typeface as the text but in a smaller font and inset from both margins, in the usual way.

My grateful thanks to Lindy Dugard who took the time to send me her latest multicultural information with her permission to use pertinent material.

I thank my family. I am especially grateful for my wonderful husband, Mike. He has been particularly patient and understanding of my need to keep writing. All of our precious living children — Greg, Peter, Cate and Sarah — have had to compete with me for computer and Internet time and I thank them for tolerating their somewhat unusual mother.

I thank God for his gifts and his peace. I take inspiration from Psalm 46:1 'God is our refuge and strength: an ever-present help in trouble.'

PREFACE

'Did I do the right thing?' and 'Is there anything else I should have done?' Most midwives working with bereaved families do a very good job when they are faced with helping a family grieving the loss of a baby. This book sets out to affirm and reassure you, whilst verifying your knowledge and giving you guidelines for 'best practice'. My hope is that you may also acquire a new perspective from information that may either be new to you or that you haven't previously considered.

When a baby dies it is not possible to have a set of procedures for management of a given condition that will lead to an expected outcome, i.e. '3 cuddles of dead baby + photos = good experience'. People are different and what will work well for one couple may not work at all for another. Using actual words from bereaved families as well as from the literature, and drawing from my own experiences, I have attempted to provide you with a range of choices in any given situation in order to foster your own creativity to enable you to individualise care for each bereaved family.

The Midwife and the Bereaved Family is divided into areas of chronological loss and subdivided into smaller sections with subheadings. It is my intention that the reader will thereby be able to quickly find a checklist or a suggestion if needed. Midwives working in labour wards may not feel it necessary to read the early pregnancy loss section; midwives working in a gynaecology setting may not wish to read about later pregnancy loss. However, I do encourage you to read all sections of this book, whether or not they address your particular area of practice, as you may gain an insight into the range of issues that confront your colleagues.

Midwives have a uniquely important role in supporting recently bereaved families and setting them on a 'good grief' path. In-depth counselling, 'stages of bereavement' and 'tasks of mourning' usually occur later than the midwife's care. They belong rightly to practising trained grief counsellors and so are not found in this book.

Midwives are in the unique position of having seen and/or 'known' the dead baby and are therefore very important to the bereaved family. Midwives are in a position of enormous responsibility when providing bereavement care to families. How we act, what we say and what we encourage parents to do or not do, impacts on them for the rest of their lives. If bereaved parents feel they were well cared for then they will often have some positive memories of the experience. If, on the other hand, they received what they consider to be poor care then they will be distressed and angry for a long time afterwards. Helping grieving families consists of the provision of care, support and information both around the time of the death and during any subsequent pregnancy and birth.

An integral part of any midwife's care is advocacy. It is as important to be an advocate for the parents when their baby dies as at any other time. This is because the parents are temporarily unable to be their own best advocate due to the debilitating effects of the trauma they are facing.

I refer to bereaved parents or families in this book but I know that sometimes the mother is alone. I feel, however, that I should always refer to the ideal situation, letting you adapt what I say to individual variations.

I have used the word 'parent' very deliberately throughout this book. I have talked to many parents whose first baby has died and who believe that they have thereby forfeited their claim to parenthood. Many will find comfort in your reassurance that they are still in fact parents.

In writing of the baby, I have used the word 'he' and I want it to read as including 'she'. I have diverged from political correctness so that it's easier to follow whom I'm talking about ('she' will always refer to the mother) and in order to avoid the awkward 'he/she', the ugly 's/he' or the contrived use of 'he' and 'she' alternately.

The time bereaved parents spend with you is the very tip of the iceberg compared with the length of their grief. It is therefore important that you refer on to community resources. It may be a good idea to keep in your workplace a resource folder (which is regularly updated) with information of local support groups, funeral directors, pastors, interpreters, counsellors and community support workers who may provide support for the parents in their grief.

Many maternity hospitals now have groups of interested people who meet and discuss 'appropriate care' of parents enduring any form of pregnancy loss. Such a group may consist of midwives, nurse managers, obstetricians, chaplains, social workers, bereavement counsellors and consumers. Such a group may consider formulating protocols, care plans, checklists and information leaflets; may air ideas; and may problem solve together. My hope is that this book will become the locus for such groups. If, as a result of this book, one bereaved family's journey is positively influenced by one midwife's care then the time and effort in writing it will have been very worthwhile.

Jane Warland
Adelaide
November 1999

CHAPTER 1

EARLY PREGNANCY LOSS

Our baby didn't get too far in its development, but it counted as a person to us.

(Speraw, 1994)

In this chapter I consider spontaneous early pregnancy loss rather than elective termination of a pregnancy.

Although there are similarities between miscarriage and elective abortion, especially in the grief following, there are also a whole range of different issues involved. Midwives are not often involved in the parents' decision to abort their baby or in follow-up of these parents. This is usually the domain of the social worker. Frequently the abortion itself is carried out with the mother as an outpatient in a day surgery unit, with little or no contact with midwives. On the other hand, midwives working in antenatal clinics, emergency departments, antenatal/gynaecological wards and labour wards all come into regular contact with women experiencing spontaneous early pregnancy loss.

DEFINITION

The term 'miscarriage' is usually understood to mean

> the spontaneous abortion of a pregnancy prior to the 20th week of pregnancy. Most miscarriages occur in the first trimester with chromosomal abnormalities (mostly aneuploidy) accounting for approximately 50% of fetal losses in the first 8-15 weeks of gestation. (Daniely et al., 1998)

A note about threatened miscarriage

Women experiencing a threatened miscarriage often live through a time of limbo lasting several days or weeks. They may be subjected to repeated blood tests and ultrasound examinations with no guarantees that the pregnancy is ongoing. Parents may feel helpless and experience a sense of powerlessness that is frequently disturbing, especially for those who are experiencing such feelings for the first time in their lives. During this time, midwives can provide information on the most likely outcome. For some this can be a time of anticipatory grieving. If the pregnancy continues, parents may find they need to adjust to the fact that the pregnancy seems to be going again. If the pregnancy ends then parents are often traumatised by their inability to be able to do anything active to prevent their baby's loss. Midwives need to be aware of the kind of trauma that these parents often endure.

Ectopic pregnancy

All of the information outlined in this chapter is also applicable to women suffering ectopic pregnancy. However women with an ectopic pregnancy often have a question mark placed over their future fertility. Furthermore, they also often face a very serious threat to their health. Therefore women with ectopic pregnancy may need especially sensitive care.

INTRODUCTION

In many emergency departments around the world miscarriage is an everyday occurrence. Most emergency departments are very busy and usually understaffed. Thus, when a woman presents who needs support and individual attention, it may be very difficult for staff to provide the support she needs.

Miscarriage can be both emotionally and physically traumatic for many women. Some women will be very afraid, some will even fear for their lives. However, there will also be a small group of women for whom a miscarriage is not perceived as a tragic event at all and who may well even welcome the end of a pregnancy about which they may have felt ambivalent. It is therefore essential that midwives not assume that this event will, or indeed will not, be emotionally traumatic for every woman for whom they care. Determining the significance of the miscarriage for the individual woman is important. Women who do not perceive their miscarriage as significant may need to be provided with different written information which downplays or omits information about coping with distress or grief, as not to do so may lead them to perceive their lack of expected response as uncaring or in some way unusual. Checklists can be printed on different coloured paper to alert staff to what has occurred without labelling the patient.

The midwifery management following is 'best practice' for couples for whom the miscarriage is perceived as a significant life event.

Preceding events

> *I was home alone when the bleeding started. Initially it was just a few drops but soon turned into a flood. I called my husband home from work and by the time he arrived I was bleeding really badly. I couldn't imagine that the baby would have survived this (but was still hopeful that it had) and started to wonder if I would make it.*

Midwives need to be aware of some of the preceding events which may lead to parents presenting with a miscarriage or threatened miscarriage. In the previous few hours the woman may have been alone and afraid. Her partner may have been called home suddenly from work. Both may be shocked and distressed by what is happening. It is therefore important that the midwife presents a calm, assured demeanour for this couple.

Organising the scan

Most miscarriages are confirmed by ultrasound scan. Midwives can assist parents by ensuring:
- the woman is not sent alone to be scanned
  (she will need support at this time)
- the sonographer is fully aware of the history
  (i.e. check that the ultrasound request form has good accurate information)
- the couple can see the ultrasound image screen for themselves
- the couple are given a 'flimsy' (ultrasound photo) of the remains of their baby
- the couple are given a copy of the ultrasound report in plain language.

BREAKING BAD NEWS

The bad news is best given, simply and honestly, as soon as the health professionals involved are aware themselves. If at all possible the doctor should tell the couple together, so that they can provide support for each other. It is important that they are made aware that there is virtually nothing that can be done to save their baby. Many times parents can feel disappointed and even angry at what they may understand as lack of medical treatment. It is crucial that they understand fully that medical science has not advanced far enough to save their tiny baby. Such information may calm their fears and relieve disappointment at perceived lack of active medical management.

Information can be given in both spoken and written form and should include:
- the usual causes of miscarriage
- any problems the miscarriage may cause to the woman both now and in the future.

Thought can be given to delivering the news in as private a setting as possible, i.e. a room with a door rather than a corridor or cubicle.

The impact of medical language on the woman and her partner or support people can be off-putting. Avoid medical terms such as 'spontaneous abortion', 'products of conception' and 'fetus' in favour of the words 'miscarriage', 'remains of the baby' and 'baby'. Wheeler (1994) states that

> when health care professionals use medical terminology to describe experiences of loss women and their family members may feel they are being treated in a cold impersonal manner that lacks sensitivity.

Although many miscarriages occur as a result of a chromosomal defect, parents often find it difficult to cope with the idea that they have produced a 'malformed' baby and may not be helped by explanations such as 'It is nature's way of getting rid of an imperfect baby'.

Some parents may doubt the accuracy of the ultrasound and be fearful that their baby is still all right. It may be possible to reassure such parents by repeating the scan using a different sonographer.

SUPPORT AFTER BAD NEWS IS BROKEN

> Miscarriage is usually an unpleasant, undignified, distressing, confusing experience. (Stead, 1996)

How can we help to make the miscarriage experience less unpleasant, undignified and distressing? Meeting expressed needs may be one way.

Stead (1996) compiled a list from Moulder (1990) and SANDS (Stillborn and Neonatal Death Society) (1991) identifying the needs of a miscarrying woman as:

- the need for care that is responsive to women's individual feelings and needs
- the need for physical care
- the need for psychological care
- the need for information
- the need for clear, sensitive and honest communication
- the need for respect and dignity
- the need for acknowledgement and legitimisation

The need for care that is responsive to women's individual feelings and needs

It is ideal to provide a 'dedicated' area for women enduring early pregnancy loss. Such consideration would show these women that their special needs are being taken into account.

After bad news is broken most parents need support, e.g. privacy, use of a telephone away from the public eye, assistance with travel and contacting partners or family and friends.

It is very important for the woman to have someone with her; if her partner is unavailable and the midwife is too busy to stay with her then a hospital chaplain or social worker may be called.

The need for physical care

It is also important that the midwife monitor the woman's physical condition, especially if she is bleeding actively, in order to avoid hypovolaemia and shock. The mother's blood group should be ascertained and Anti-D/Rhogam administered if necessary.

Parents may also appreciate a warm beverage (provided the woman is not fasting for surgery!) analgesia or a sedative to take home, provision of sanitary pads or protective pads if bleeding is heavy, tissues, and a cool face washer.

The need for psychological care

Most bereaved parents appreciate the opportunity to talk after receiving bad news. This is not the time for in-depth counselling; it is the time for listening and providing understanding. When you are with the couple, it is important not to make assumptions about the impact of the miscarriage. Listen as the parents divulge what is happening to them emotionally, acknowledge their loss, give them permission to cry and provide them with comfort if they are crying.

Most parents would appreciate your sitting with them rather than standing over them.

The need for information

Moulder (1990) found that providing information to the couple was very important, second only to the understanding shown by staff. Information needs to include: what has happened, what is happening now and what might happen next, as well as suggestions about why it might be happening.

When giving information the following issues are important:
- Give accurate information and communicate it clearly, honestly, promptly, at appropriate times and in an unbiased, unhurried manner.
- Include information about practical matters, such as procedures and arrangements.
- Be specific, e.g. how much bleeding to expect; how much bleeding is a matter of concern; and when, how and who to contact in cases of concern.
- If possible, offer a range of choices.
- Answer all questions.
- Avoid no subject.
- Give information that is consistent. (It is important to restrict the numbers of professionals providing information so as not to confuse or overwhelm the couple.)

It is also important to explain what will happen next and the reasons for any delays. Parents need to be offered choices about what happens next. This may help them re-establish a sense of control.

The need for clear, sensitive and honest communication

Give the bereaved parents time to consider their options: a 'medical miscarriage' or a D&C (dilatation and curettage) — give the parents written and spoken information about what to expect from each. It is important to repeat information several times in several different ways and to offer the options over and over.

D&C: If a D&C is decided upon, the woman will need written as well as spoken information on:
• how long the surgery will take
• what anaesthetic is involved
• what analgesia she will require
• when she will be fit to go home
• how long it will take to recuperate physically once she is home.

Medical miscarriage: If the couple choose to have a medical miscarriage they need to be told the most likely sequelae, prior to departure from hospital:
• how long the woman is liable to bleed
• how much bleeding is 'normal'
• how much bleeding is 'too much'.

A medical miscarriage may involve a 'mini' labour. Women need to be prepared for this as contractions and the delivery of a baby may be an unexpected trauma if it was expected that the baby would just 'slip out', with little or no discomfort. Enduring pain and discomfort when there is no joy at the end may be an unexpected trauma.

Mothers often wonder if they will be able to recognise their tiny baby in the tissue they pass. Midwives may need to describe what is likely to be seen. (Many parents do not expect to see a perfectly formed little baby which is often what is seen in a late miscarriage.)

Make sure the attending doctor communicates with the referring GP, especially if follow-up appointments are to be made with the GP. It is advisable to make the initial follow-up appointment before the couple leaves the hospital.

Parents need to know who to contact if they are concerned and an alternative contact if that person is unavailable.

The need for respect and dignity
As midwives we tread a very fine line between giving the couple the privacy they need and leaving them alone so that they feel deserted.

It is almost always appropriate to give a couple some time alone, ideally in a room with a door rather than a cubicle with a curtain. If it is at all possible avoid leaving the woman on a trolley in a corridor or other public place and definitely do not ask her to change into a hospital gown unless you are sure she is going to the operating theatres immediately.

It is particularly important for a woman who is miscarrying that care is taken to minimise her distress by making pelvic examinations as short as possible, and by maintaining privacy and respect with minimal interruptions whilst the examinations are taking place. Even something as simple as knocking on a door or asking if you can come in gives a sense of control back to the woman, who may feel as though everything that is happening to her is out of her control. Other ways to give back a sense of control are to encourage parents to make choices about aspects of their care:

- when or if a D&C will occur
- whether a pathology examination will occur
- how the fetus will be disposed of
- whether there will be mementoes and a memorial service.

People far from home may need special consideration as to their requirements for accommodation or support.

Staff should ascertain the safety of either one of the couple leaving the hospital alone. Try to detain the person until transport arrives.

The need for acknowledgement and legitimisation

Do not offer clichés such as 'you can always have another', 'it is nature's way' or 'time heals'. These may be true but it is never helpful to hear any of them immediately after a loss. Instead, say 'I'm sorry' or 'Would you like to talk about it?'

> Carers who make comments rationalising the loss to parents may be perceived as uncaring. Nurses need to be tactful and be aware that chance remarks may be taken out of context and exaggerated if they touch a raw nerve. (Stead, 1996)

As midwives we must be careful not to intimate that this precious baby can be replaced, by saying or implying that the parents can easily have another. None of us would suggest it is appropriate that a newly bereaved widow get another husband and yet it is common for newly bereaved parents to be treated this way.

Your own reaction

It is important for health care providers to be aware that the means of coping that they use to shield themselves from emotional pain (so that they can continue to practice effectively) may actually cause significant distress in the patients they seek to help. The challenge before providers, therefore, is to practice in a way that clearly communicates understanding and compassion without crossing over a personal boundary that would lead to over-involvement. (Speraw, 1994)

In caring for miscarrying women we need to be careful about our own feelings and how we communicate these to the bereaved parents. We need to be mindful about what we say and how we say it. Bereaved parents are often highly sensitised to honesty. Therefore we need to be honest about expressing our feelings. We might be tempted to minimise the effect that a miscarriage can have on a young teenage mother, or a grand-multiparous mother, and feel more for the couple who have just miscarried after years of infertility. However, every couple deserves treatment that is compassionate and appropriate to their loss as they perceive it. If you feel sorry that their baby has died then it is appropriate to say, 'I'm sorry your baby has died'. If you don't feel especially sad for a particular couple, then perhaps saying something like 'I realise this must be a difficult time for you right now' may be more appropriate than saying you feel sorry if you do not.

Admission to hospital

If a woman needs to be admitted to hospital, prior to her admission she needs to be made aware of how long she is likely to stay, the type of hospital accommodation that is available and the most likely scenarios for her case.

Parents need to be aware that they may meet women who have had or are preparing for a termination of pregnancy. Avoid putting such women in the same room. As one woman found:

When I woke up from the anaesthetic I found myself sharing a room with a young woman who asked me how far along I was. She assumed that I was there for the same reason as her, an elective abortion. I couldn't get out of the room quick enough. It was pretty insensitive of the staff to do that to me.

CHECKLIST FOR MIDWIFERY CARE IN MISCARRIAGE AND ECTOPIC PREGNANCY

You may find the following checklist (adapted from Wheeler, 1994: 225) useful in helping those mothers who require surgical intervention after an early pregnancy loss. Take some time to adapt the list to suit your hospital.

Telephone the patient 24 hours before admission or perform this assessment upon admission to perioperative area.
- Assess the patient's perception of her loss.
- Assess the patient's coping strategies.
- Tell her about the hospital's admission procedures and what to expect during surgery.

Keep family members together as much as possible.

Prepare the operating room.
- Cover the instruments.
- Cover the suction machine or place it out of sight.
- Conceal the stirrups until anaesthesia is induced.

Offer options based on your assessment of the patient.
- Notify the person in charge of pastoral care to be ready for a blessing or naming ceremony or some kind of memorial service.
- Show the family pictures of normal fetal development.
- Show the family the remains of the baby, but only if you have obtained permission first.
- Find out what the family wants to do with the remains of the baby (e.g. cremation or burial, by the hospital or by the family).
- Give the patient written material on miscarriage or ectopic pregnancy (whichever is relevant) and on grief responses.

Follow the patient up after she is discharged.
- Telephone her within 24 hours, then at one week and at six weeks.
- Refer the patient (and perhaps the family) to a local support group.
- Coordinate the patient's care with the obstetric care provider's office.

Meeting the baby

I asked the doctor if I could see what he got during the D&C, and his response was 'You don't really want to'. I wouldn't have asked if I didn't want to. I still, to this day, would have liked to see what he got from me. (Wheeler, 1994)

It is important to be open to queries from bereaved parents. Many parents express the desire to have the opportunity to see their baby; they need to be prepared for what they may see by someone who has already looked.

It is never appropriate to show the remains of the baby to a parent without asking their permission first. One woman woke from anaesthetic following a D&C to be confronted by the remains of her baby, in a specimen jar, by her bed. She successfully sued the hospital for putting her through such trauma.

Midwives need to ask parents if they want to see the remains of their baby whether it is indeterminate tissue or a tiny fetus. (It may be possible with a later spontaneous miscarriage to clean and wrap the baby for the parents to see.) Some tiny babies may need to be nestled in the palm of your hand or perhaps a sea shell of suitable size and shape. A tiny fetus may be able to be wrapped in a gauze swab. Dolls' baskets of different sizes may be used to show the baby to the parents. It is completely inappropriate to show the parents their baby in a kidney dish, bed-pan or specimen jar.

Determine from the parents whether baptism is desired for their fetus and organise a minister of religion to be present. In circumstances where baptism of the fetus is not possible, parents may wish to formally 'name' or 'dedicate' their baby.

Helping to create memories

When a baby dies under 20 weeks, it is rare that concrete mementoes (photos, handprints, footprints) will be able to be collected easily at the time of the loss. Therefore many families do not have any tangible evidence that their baby existed. Some may want proof. It may be appropriate to offer a letter or certificate to prove that the pregnancy really happened.

As a midwife, if you initiate, support and encourage parents to create memories, they may feel able to continue creating memories after they leave hospital. Use your creativity to help bereaved parents create memories of their baby that are meaningful and enriching to them. Perhaps you could make some suggestions from the Early Pregnancy Loss Memory Creation List.

EARLY PREGNANCY LOSS MEMORY CREATION LIST FOR PARENTS

- Keep the positive pregnancy test. (This test may be taken after fetal demise whilst pregnancy hormones are still present.)
- Keep an ultrasound picture (but note that ultrasound 'flimsies' are destroyed if they are laminated).
- Choose a flower to remember the baby by, perhaps a flower blooming at the time of the baby's death. Buy that flower at anniversary times. Include the flower in family portraits to symbolise your baby's presence.
- Precious stones are associated with months of the year. Buy a piece of jewellery with a stone appropriate to the baby's date of birth or due date.
- Select something which symbolises the baby, perhaps an angel, a cherub, a butterfly or a star. Buy jewellery with the baby's symbol on it to remember the baby.
- Use the baby's due date or birth date for personal identification numbers or access codes. You will remember the baby every time you use the code.
- Name the baby. Naming helps you focus on the person rather than the event. In the future you can say 'when I had John' rather than 'when I had the miscarriage'. If the baby's sex is unknown you may consider using a special family name, a name already chosen for the gender you had hoped for or a unisex name.
- Buy a large candle with the baby's name on it. This can be lit on special occasions — birthdays, mother's day, father's day, Christmas etc. — and the baby will be included in the celebration.
- Each year buy an age-appropriate ornament for the Christmas tree or an age-appropriate gift for the child and then, perhaps, donate it to a charity.
- A crystal vase with the baby's birth date or due date engraved on it can be used each year for flowers on that day.
- Plant a tree or bush.
- Press or dry any flowers received from family and friends.
- Buy the paper of the day of the birth date or due date. Most newspapers have archives and a copy may be obtained from them.

- Keep any cards received.
- Place a memorial notice in the newspaper every year then cut the notices out and keep them.
- Create a baby box for cards, dried flowers, notices, etc.
- Donate a book or video to the hospital, the SANDS (Stillbirth and Neonatal Death Support) library or other library in memory of the baby.
- Find out if the hospital has a chapel. Regular services may be held for bereaved people to come to remember their loved one. Some hospitals also have a remembrance book which can be signed in memory of a loved one of whatever age.

Family-focused care

Speraw (1994) found in her study of 40 couples that both parents experience the loss. Men may appear to be strong, coping and supportive of their partner but under all that facade is a grieving male probably feeling helpless, vulnerable and fearful of losing a wife as well as a child while being powerless to save them. Speraw (1994: 214) says:

> With each person immersed in his or her own grief, the couple may not know how to support each other. It is the role of the health professional to help prepare couples for the differences in grief they may see in each other. They should be encouraged to talk about their feelings of loss and sadness.

Ideally the woman's partner should be allowed to stay with her while she is undergoing the miscarriage.

Couples need to know that it is usual for each to grieve differently. Encourage them to keep the lines of communication open.

> If a father doesn't share his thoughts and emotions, and conveys the message to his wife that he believes her need to talk about their child's death is obsessive ('dwelling on it', morbid, or self-indulgent), then the communication gap between them will broaden, and the grief process will become an even more intensely disturbing experience for both of them. (Staudacher, 1991)

Refer parents to a self-help group such as SANDS, Bonnie Babes, or Compassionate Friends. Just prior to discharge, give the couple contact details and pamphlets and say something like 'You may not need this information now but you may want to refer to it in the next couple of weeks'.

Information for children at home

Young children are more perceptive than many people believe. If the couple have children at home, it may be appropriate to recommend good reading material for them and make some suggestions about telling them clearly and simply what happened to their expected sibling.

POST-DISCHARGE SUPPORT

On discharge from the hospital tell the bereaved parents of the kind of things to expect and give them the information in writing as well. Topics that need to be covered include:

- what to expect on arrival at home
- emotional recovery
- dealing with physical symptoms such as fatigue, bleeding, signs of infection or retained products
- contraception.

Give them a list of people to contact and suggested times for contacting them, e.g. their GP, the hospital social worker, any local support groups.

Perhaps discuss with the couple how to handle clichés from well-meaning family and friends. One simple reply may be 'Thanks for trying to help but that is *not* how I feel.'

The fact of the pregnancy may not have been widely known. The mother may therefore be embarrassed to mention that she was pregnant. This means the woman often grieves her loss privately and a sense of isolation may result.

Midwives need to acknowledge parents' feelings. Tell the parents not to expect their grief to resolve quickly.

Follow-up

Coordination of follow-up between the obstetric care provider and the midwife will enable the couple to receive good care. If the obstetric caregiver is aware of what was offered to the couple during their hospital stay it will be easier to follow up on the couple's care at the six-week check. The six-week postnatal check usually includes:

- a discussion of pathology findings (a plain language report may be given to the family)
- a physical check
- an emotional check
- a discussion on contraception and subsequent pregnancy plans.

It is usually appreciated if the midwife makes a follow-up telephone call at predictably difficult times (e.g. within the first week, six weeks later, at the due date, at the one-year anniversary). This lets the woman and her family know that they are still remembered. These calls provide opportunities for the family to:

- ask questions
- share their feelings
- seek advice
- request particulars about the process of grief
- obtain information about local support groups.

A nice touch that one hospital uses is to write a letter of sympathy to the couple which is sent to them after discharge. This is a practice which may be emulated. It is usually welcomed by the parents receiving the letter.

Saying goodbye

> ... we would like to put on record our belief that on general ethical grounds of respect, all mothers ... should be given the opportunity clearly to express their wishes about the eventual disposal of the dead fetus, and that these wishes should, wherever possible, be respected. (Polkinghorne Report, in Kohner, 1992)

Many parents wish to know what will happen to the remains of their baby. Some will be distressed to find out later that their baby was disposed of in the hospital incinerator and may have preferred to have been given the option to take their baby home for burial.

Ownership of the baby can become an issue. Parents may wish to exercise the option of taking their baby home either before or after pathology tests.

It is wise not to make assumptions about parents' wishes regarding a funeral for their baby. While a formal funeral is not a legal requirement for a baby born dead before the stipulated age of viability (20 weeks), some parents feel that they need this chance to say goodbye to their baby.

Many hospitals are becoming aware of this issue and some are keeping fetal remains to be cremated together and sprinkled at a certain place. Parents then have the opportunity to visit such a place and remember their baby. Parents need to be aware that there may be no 'ashes' available after cremation of a tiny fetus. This is because the temperature is such that the baby evaporates, leaving no remains.

Some hospitals can arrange for a burial or cremation through an undertaker even if the baby is not 'entitled' to a funeral. Parents may have to bear the cost of the interment.

A remembrance service may be organised where parents can create a meaningful memory of what their baby meant to them. This can be done many months or even years after the baby's death.

One hospital keeps track of the baby and what is happening in each case by using a triplicate 'tracking' system form — one part is filed in the patient's notes, one part goes with the baby and the other goes to the doctor's office. This form includes the items 'chosen mode of disposal' and 'funeral arrangements' (Kohner, 1992).

As midwives we need to:
- be able to offer parents a respectful and dignified disposal for their baby's remains
- have information about disposal options which we can pass on to parents.
- know individual hospitals' procedures in relation to storage and disposal of babies' remains
- offer parents time to decide — this means there must be accurate labelling, documentation and storage of the baby
- be proactive in changing inappropriate hospital procedure to an acceptable standard. (Adapted from Kohner, 1992)

REFERENCES

Daniely M, Aviram-Goldring A, Barkai G, Goldman B (1998): Detection of chromosomal aberration in fetuses arising from recurrent spontaneous abortion by comparative genomic hybridization. *Hum Reprod.* 13 (4) April: 805–809.

Kohner N (1992): *A Dignified Ending.* London: SANDS

Moulder C (1990): *Miscarriage: Women's Experiences and Needs.* London: Pandora

SANDS (Stillbirth and Neonatal Death Support) (1991): *Miscarriage, Stillbirth and Neonatal Death — guidelines for professionals.* London: SANDS.

Speraw S (1994): The experience of miscarriage: How couples define quality in health care delivery. *Journal of Perinatology* 14 (3): 208–215.

Staudacher C (1991): *Men and Grief.* Oakland: New Harbinger.

Stead CE (1996): Nursing management in the Accident and Emergency department of women undergoing a miscarriage. *Accident and Emergency Nursing* 4: 182–186.

Wheeler S (1994): Psychosocial needs of women during miscarriage or ectopic pregnancy. *AORN Journal* 60 (2) August: 221–231.

INTERESTING RESEARCH ARTICLES

Bansen S, Stevens HA (1992): Women's experiences of miscarriage in early pregnancy. *Journal of Nurse-Midwifery:* 37 (2): 84–90.

Conway K (1991): Miscarriage *J of Psychosomatic Obs & Gynae:*12: 121–131.

Cormell M (1992): Just another miscarriage? *Nursing Times* 88 (48) 25 Nov.: 41–43.

Davies M, Geoghegan J (1994): Developing an early pregnancy assessment unit. *Nursing Times* 90 (44) 2 Nov.

Henshaw RC et al. (1993): Medical management of miscarriage: non-surgical uterine evacuation of incomplete and inevitable spontaneous abortion. *BMJ* 30: 894.

Hutti MH (1988) Behavioural issues: Miscarriage — The parent's point of view. *J Emerg Nursing* 14 (6): 367–368.

Hutti M (1992): Parents' perceptions of the miscarriage experience. *Death Studies* 16: 401–415.

Koziol-McLain J (1992): An investigation of emergency department patients' perceptions of their miscarriage experience. *J of Emerg. Nursing* 18 (6) Dec.: 501–504.

Laurent C (1991): Marking the loss. *Nursing Times* 87: 26–27.

Layne L (1990): Motherhood lost: cultural dimensions of miscarriage and stillbirth in America. *Women's Health* 16: 69–98.

Ramsden C (1995): Miscarriage counselling — an accident and emergency perspective. *Accident and Emergency Nursing* 3: 68–73.

Regan L (1992): Managing miscarriage. *Practitioner* 236 (1513) Apr.: 374–8.

Roberts H (1991): Managing miscarriage: the management of the emotional sequelae of miscarriage in training practices in the west of Scotland. *Fam Prac* 8: 117–120.

Steele M (1992): Behavioural issues. The emotional trauma of miscarriage in the emergency department: A first person account. *J of Emerg Nurs* 18 (1) Feb.: 54–56.

Stewart A et al. (1992): Miscarriage *Professional Nurse* July: 656-60.

Turner M (1991): Management after spontaneous miscarriage. *BMJ* 302: 909-910.

Wells R (1991)Managing miscarriage: the need for more than medical mechanics. *Postgraduate Medicine* 89 (2): 207-212.

RECOMMENDED READING

Berezin N (1982): *After a Loss in Pregnancy, Help for Families Affected by Miscarriage, a Stillbirth or the Loss of a New-Born.* New York: Simon and Schuster.

Borg S, Lasker J (1989): *When Pregnancy Fails: Families Coping with Miscarriage, Ectopic Pregnancy, Stillbirth and Infant Death.* New York: Bantam.

Fritsch J, Ilse S (1988):*The Anguish of Loss.* Maple Plain, MN: Wintergreen Press.

Ilse S (1990) *Empty Arms: Coping with Miscarriage, Stillbirth and Infant Death.* Long Lake, MN: Wintergreen Press.

Jones W (1990): *Miscarriage* London: Thorsons

Limbo R, Wheeler S (1993): *When a Baby Dies: A Handbook for Healing and Helping.* La Crosse, WI: TRS Bereavement Services.

Luebbermann M (1995): *Coping with Miscarriage: A Simple Reassuring Guide to Emotional and Physical Healing.* Rocklin, CA: Prima Publishing.

Mander R (1994): *Loss and Bereavement in Childbearing.* Oxford: Blackwell Science.

Murray J (1993): *An Ache in Their Hearts* Resource Package. Brisbane: The University of Queensland.

Nicol M (1997): *Loss of a Baby.* Sydney: Harper Collins.

Oakley A et al. (1990): *Miscarriage.* London: Penguin Books.

Raphael-Leff J (1991): *Psychological Processes of Childbearing* London: Chapman & Hall.

Townsend R, Perkins A (1992): *A Bitter Fruit.* Alameda: Hunter House.

Vogel G (1996): *A Caregiver's Handbook To Perinatal Loss*. Minnesota: deRuyter-Nelson Publications.

CHAPTER 2

MID TRIMESTER LOSS

A closed mouth gathers no feet.

(Lette, 1996)

PREJUDICE

Whilst researching this chapter I heard many stories from families who had been subject to prejudice.

- Some families had elected to terminate their pregnancy and had subsequently suffered care from health professionals who were cool or distant towards them.
- Others had elected to continue their pregnancy in the face of a poor or hopeless diagnosis and had been subjected to reproach and misunderstanding from the health professionals assigned to their care.

Neither of these situations is acceptable. Letting your own prejudice show to families in need is completely reprehensible. It is therefore crucially important that you consider your own opinions and make a decision as to which families you can care for. If you find you cannot agree with a family's decision, it may be appropriate for you to decline to care for them or to hand their care over before you become too far involved.

PRENATAL TESTING

I had a CVS which was positive for Down syndrome. When these results came back I didn't want to believe them and we didn't know what to do. Weeks ticked by with us both in limbo. Finally we decided to have an amnio. The worst time was waiting for the amnio results. I did not want to be pregnant. I did not tell anyone about the pregnancy but I was starting to show. I did not want to eat and make the baby grow but I didn't want to take pain relief or sleeping tablets in case they harmed the baby. I couldn't sleep. I wanted time to stop until the results were back. The amnio confirmed Down Syndrome so after 19 weeks of pregnancy and 10 weeks of hell we terminated the pregnancy.

Prenatal testing is being offered to more and more women as a matter of routine but the conditions found usually cannot be treated. Therefore couples who find that they have a baby with a chromosomal error, major organ abnormalities or neural tube defect are being asked to make decisions about continuing the pregnancy or aborting.

Most parents undergo prenatal tests in the belief that the results will confirm the health of their baby. Therefore, most parents are unprepared for the consequences of such screening if they are unfortunate enough to have a baby with an abnormality. If an abnormality is found then the parents are faced with Hobson's choice.

Hobson's choice

According to the 10th edition of Webster's Dictionary (Merriam-Webster, 1998), Hobson's choice is 'an apparently free choice that offers no real alternative'. That's the 'choice' some parents feel they have.

The decision to have a mid trimester abortion was the most horrible one I have ever had to make in my life. You are faced with two very lousy choices. You can choose to carry on the pregnancy and make the best life you can for your child knowing that he will be disabled and may not have the quality of life you dreamed of for your child. Or you can choose to terminate the pregnancy you longed for. You agonise because you wonder what the child would have been like. You wonder if you are making the decision for selfish reasons (either way). Are you choosing to terminate because you are being selfish and do not want the burden of raising a disabled child? Are you choosing to continue for selfish reasons because you so desperately want this child that you don't care about his quality of life?

BREAKING BAD NEWS

This kind of news is painful and shocking regardless of how it is given or who tells you. (SAFDA, 1995)

Parents who have been in this situation have said:
• It is best to break bad news face to face. Avoid using the telephone in this instance as it can be seen as very cold and impersonal. If the use of the telephone is unavoidable, ensure the parent receiving the news is not alone.
• Gentle and thoughtful breaking of the news is appreciated.
• Ideally a person who is known to the couple should break the news.
• Try to tell both parents together. If this is not possible ensure the parent who receives the news has a support person present. This may be a member of the family, close friend, hospital social worker or chaplain.
• Explain what has gone wrong in terms that the couple can understand. Avoid medical terminology. One mother says her doctor said 'Your product of conception has a condition that is incompatible with survivability'. Her response was 'What? You mean my baby will die?'

Information and support after bad news is broken

'Your baby has anencephaly.' In just those few words, all our hopes and dreams for our longed-for child had gone up in smoke.

Be aware that parents who have received bad news may be in shock. They may suffer physical reactions — feel faint, suffer palpitations, feel nauseous, even vomit. Midwifery measures or medication may need to be considered. Above all the parents need time to think about their choices.

Offer the options over and over both in writing and verbally. Give the parents privacy. Allow them time with you, time together, time for each to think separately if they wish.

Offer to help them seek a second opinion — parents can doubt what is being said, especially as antenatal testing can be inaccurate. (Julian Reynier et al., 1994; Clayton-Smith et al., 1990; Griffiths et al., 1996)

Make appointments with health/helping professionals or support groups to help the parents in their decision making. Encourage them to write down any questions they have. These might cover the following topics (SAFDA, 1995):
- the likely range of ability and disability associated with the disorder
- the likely quality of life for the baby and family
- any expected breakthroughs in treatment for the disorder
- implications for future pregnancies
- any maternal risks associated with the abnormality found in the baby
- all the options, support, alternatives and choices available.

Tell the couple when results of any further tests will be available and explain any likely reasons for delay.

Think about your language. Malformed or not the baby is still the parents' longed-for child. There is a difference between saying 'you have a spina bifida baby' and 'your baby has spina bifida.'

It is also important to explain that the baby will probably be perfectly formed apart from the defect/s. It is especially important to explain that a hydrocephalic baby may not have a monstrously big head, as parents of such babies may believe there has been some mistake if an apparently normal baby is born after a genetic termination.
One mother said:

> Everybody had told me that I couldn't have done anything to cause the problems. I believed their hearts were in the right place and they didn't want me to suffer from guilt, but I didn't believe them. How could these people know? They didn't know what I had done from day to day throughout my pregnancy, only I did. Hearing that I couldn't have **prevented** the problems no matter what I did seemed valid since it would encompass everything I did during my pregnancy. (Grady and O'Leary, 1993)

Explanations can also be offered about what it is that the parents are really being offered. Provide written information, either about the condition the baby has or where the parents can obtain more information. Encourage the parents to get in touch with other parents who have children with the particular disability.

Prepare the parents for how they are likely to feel towards the pregnancy; feelings of alienation and repulsion are common and may be frightening, as one mother explained:

> *I didn't want to touch my stomach for days. I felt alienated,*
> *even a little repulsed, by the movements of that baby that had*
> *filled me with such joy the day before I heard the news. It was*
> *a terrible time.*

Be aware that whatever else you can do for this family, you do not make the decision about what happens next for them. They and only they must make the decision and then they must live with their decision with your care and support.

Waters and Richardson (1998) suggest that the parents' decision will be influenced by some or many of the following factors:

* belief systems
* treatment for the disorder
* previous life events
* family resources, e.g. finances and physical support available
* family dynamics, such as impact on other children of the family, the partner and their relationship.

The authors further state that there are many external pressures including:

* pressure to make a decision based on often groundless time constraints
* pressure to make a decision before 20 weeks' gestation, without allowing the parents enough time to make the decision that is right for them
* pressure to make a decision quickly, based on an opinion that this is 'best' for the parents or even 'best for all concerned'
* pressure which causes the partner to fear for the woman's life if the pregnancy continues, where no medical risk is evident.
* the pressure of being pressured to make a decision.

CLINICAL MANAGEMENT

(when parents elect to interrupt the pregnancy)

I was told that the standard medical therapy for this condition was 'early delivery'. I would have a laminaria tent placed inside my cervix and would be smeared with a prostaglandin gel. This would start my labour and could take 24–72 hours to complete, and would give me a fever, vomiting, diarrhoea, and the shakes. I would deliver a small fetus that I could hold and bury if I wished.

It is important that parents are informed about (SAFDA, 1995):
- what to expect to feel before, during, and after the procedure
- the types of procedures used to interrupt a pregnancy
- the risks, side effects and possible complications of each procedure
- likely time frames for procedures
- whether they have a choice of procedure
- pain relief options
- how the baby will be after birth
- seeing and spending time with the baby after birth
- the care of the baby afterward, e.g. photographing, need for post-mortem
- the guidelines for birth/death certificates
- funeral arrangements/memorial service
- the partner or other support person remaining with the mother throughout the stay
- all aspects of care while in hospital
- legal considerations.

WHERE

Some hospitals have a policy for women undergoing genetic termination to give birth in the gynaecology area rather than the labour ward. However, it is preferable in most instances to use the labour ward, as most gynaecology areas are not well set up for women giving birth. Delivery away from a busy, noisy labour ward can still be a choice offered to all couples undergoing genetic termination.

LABOUR AND BIRTH

Be aware that it is:
- common for the parents to have second thoughts
- appropriate to initiate antenatal counselling
- advisable to encourage the parents to read about all the options available so that informed choice may be employed.
- germane to encourage parents to write a birth plan
- necessary that all health professionals caring for the couple are nonjudgmental regarding the parents' decision
- appropriate to inform parents of the likely scenarios surrounding induced termination, i.e. fever, chills, diarrhoea, nausea, vomiting etc.

MEETING THE BABY

> *He was born alive and my husband and I held him in our arms for the 20 minutes his tiny heart beat. We cried the entire time and told him how much we loved him. I was afraid to look at his abnormalities but what I can now only really remember seeing is his sweet little nose and lovely little fingers and toes. It wasn't nearly as bad as I thought it would be.*

Parents may have no idea what to expect when they see their baby. It is natural that they may be afraid to look at and cuddle their baby.

Wrap the baby in a warm blanket. Describe the baby first, then introduce the baby. Hold the baby yourself, stroke and talk to the baby using his name, then slowly approach the parents with the baby in your arms. If the parents remain unsure put their hands over yours.

Often parents will take their cue from you. How you handle and speak of the baby will be watched and, in many cases, emulated by parents.

Gross abnormality should not preclude contact. Encourage parents to have contact with their baby by looking first yourself and then giving them a description of what you see, always remembering to start with positive comments. Point out the baby's normal features then give the parents an explanation of the abnormality. Let them investigate the abnormality when they feel ready to do so.

When encouraging parents to see their patently abnormal baby tell them that, if they look, what they are most likely to remember will be their baby's perfect features. If they don't look they are likely to live with their imagination of what the abnormality looked like and they won't have the other memories to offset their imagination. As one mother said:

> *His tiny head was extremely enlarged and disfigured due to the hydrocephalus. His tiny back had a hole exposing his spinal column and spinal nerves. But still I thought of him only as beautiful.*

Small, fragile babies may be wrapped in a lightweight cloth such as muslin. Attempting to dress the baby may lead to damage and is best left to a mortician.

Indicate gender only if you are certain. Be especially cautious if the genitalia are ambiguous or the baby is very immature. Don't offer an opinion unless you can have it confirmed by another experienced midwife then document it in the medical record. If parents are given an incorrect gender there can be quite disastrous psychological consequences for them when the autopsy results show a different gender.

> *No-one was completely sure what sex our baby was and so we had to wait for the autopsy results (24 hours) to find out. It was a horrible wait but still preferable to being told the wrong thing.*

It is important for parents to be reminded prior to discharge that they can see their baby again if they wish. It is especially important to make this offer if they have chosen not to see their baby, as this mother found:

> My social worker said she'd bring him back later if I wanted to and I still said 'NO, no no'... and of course I got home and I had lots of time to think about it and I just assumed he'd be gone, that everything would be finalised. But she rang and she said 'Timothy's still here'... so we came in and had a lovely cuddle and a hold ... It was 7 days later, you need that time ... you need some space. (SAFDA, 1995)

SAYING GOODBYE

Babies born prior to 20 weeks' gestation (later in some countries) do not require a funeral. However many parents may wish their baby to be buried or cremated. It may be particularly difficult for parents who have interrupted a pregnancy to decide what they want to do about their baby's remains. Some parents choose to leave the hospital still wondering whether to hold a funeral. Reassure them that their baby will be kept in the hospital mortuary until they make a decision.

DISCHARGE PLANNING

Going home is almost always difficult for the parents. It is helpful for discharge information to be written as well as spoken. Discharge planning may include the following kinds of information.

- Tell the parents where the baby will be and whether they will still be able to visit after they go home.
- Introduce them to local support agencies or other support people. Provide information about who to contact if they need to talk, including self-help support groups as well as social workers, chaplains etc.
- Warn them of likely reactions from family and friends. Some bereaved parents may find their family and friends are judgmental about their decision to terminate the pregnancy because of a genetically abnormal baby. Genetic termination is often an emotive issue. It may be wise to counsel the bereaved parents to be selective about confiding in their friends.
- Alert bereaved mothers, before they leave hospital, to the fact that loss in the second trimester may be accompanied by the need to suppress lactation. Some lactation suppression tips are given in the next chapter.
- Let parents know there will be bad days for some time after their baby's loss. The reason for a bad day may not be apparent immediately, as this mother found:

> *I had a really bad day 3 months after her death and couldn't figure out why until I realised that this was the day I was supposed to give up work to make some last minute preparations for the baby. Instead I was already back at work without the baby. No-one knew the significance of the day but it was very painful for me.*

FOLLOW-UP

Parents who have endured a genetic termination should be 'followed-up' after about two weeks for emotional and physical assessment as well as at six weeks for a postnatal check which includes discussion of autopsy findings, recurrence risks and referral for genetic counselling. It is good to write a letter to the couple's GP to include information about the six-week assessment, relevant further investigations, referrals and suggestions for management of future pregnancies.

CLINICAL MANAGEMENT

(when parents elect to continue the pregnancy)

We debated for about 5 minutes — I confess it seemed like we should go ahead and induce because the child would die anyway. Why go through a difficult pregnancy when we knew that the outcome was certain death? I was ambivalent about being pregnant, but then I realised that this was my child, growing within me, and she deserved just as much love as my other two. Why would I turn my back on her just because she was missing an organ? If my other two lost a limb, or an organ, I wouldn't love them any less.

I think that my doctor was upset and scared by our decision to carry our baby to term. I know that he had never dealt with this before and was feeling frightened and not completely on top of this. I also think he lacked any emotional skills to help me carry this child, and felt that it would be easier on everyone if we would just terminate.

(Mother of a baby with a prenatal diagnosis of anencephaly)

The following issues (drawn from SAFDA, 1995) need to be discussed and decisions must be made, with all parties agreeing to what will happen:

- How will the baby be after birth?
- Is the baby likely to die at or after birth?
- Will the baby need surgery soon after birth?
- What input do the parents have in the medical management of the baby?
- Can the parents make decisions about whether to proceed with life-saving measures?
- What resources are available to families with a special-needs child?
- How can we access services?

WHAT NEXT?

Parents may wish to take time during the remainder of the pregnancy to prepare for their baby's birth and/or death. Here are some issues that they may wish to consider, together with comments from parents who have been in similar situations.

- **Choosing their baby's place of birth:**
  I chose a home birth because I wanted her to be surrounded by people who loved her. I didn't feel that I could control that in a hospital setting, and if she was only going to live a few minutes, I wanted them to be wonderful minutes.

- **Making decisions about the involvement of surviving children:**
  The plan was to involve all the children. The baby was as much their brother as our son. They needed to be able to say their hellos and their goodbyes too.

- **Choosing the baby's name:**
  Because we had had an amnio we knew the baby's sex. We decided on 'Peter', we knew he would need to be a 'rock' to cling to his life after he was born.

- **Baptism:**
  We organised a priest to stand by to baptise him immediately he was born

- **Planning a funeral and/or a memorial service:**
  I felt an urgency to take control of whatever I could — collecting pictures of anencephalic babies, planning the birth, the funeral, anything to make me feel in control of this totally out-of-control situation

- **What keepsakes and/or photos they wish to have:**
  We made moulds of his feet. We counted his toes and fingers. He was a perfect baby in every other aspect.

- **How to contact appropriate support groups both for the specified abnormality and/or for bereavement support**

- **Planning the birth announcement** — here is how one family announced the birth of their baby:

Dear Family and Friends

Sean is a very special baby, and the birth announcement can't possibly say it all. God has made Sean special and chosen us to be his parents — we feel blessed. Sean was born with Down syndrome. We want to give you time to adjust to the news, so you won't feel the need to have an immediate response. We hope you will feel the same as we do, we're happy and proud. We would like you to see him as we do, a beautiful baby boy. We also want you to treat him just like any other baby — congratulate us. We have a baby, we're a family now. This is not a sad moment. PLEASE do not apologise, we aren't sorry. We are still gathering information on Down syndrome and probably won't be able to answer any questions for a while. We would like to encourage you to call on us — come to see Sean. He sleeps, eats, cries and dirties diapers, just like every other baby, he's just got an extra chromosome.

COPING WITH THE REMAINDER OF THE PREGNANCY

Physically I was now my baby's intensive care unit for the next six months.

Coping with the remainder of the pregnancy in the face of fetal diagnosis, especially if the prognosis is poor or it is known that the baby will die, has been described by parents as a very stressful yet somehow fulfilling time. One mother says of this time:

> *The next months were just like living with a child with a terminal diagnosis. Eric had a condition that would take his life, and we had an approximate date when this would occur. Just like parents of terminally ill children, I cherished this time I had with him. I knew that as long as he was in the womb, he would be all right. His strong kicks and constant activity were a reminder that his life was strong. He didn't know there was anything wrong with him.*

PLANNING FOR THE BIRTH

> *On booking into hospital, I informed the midwife of my condition and found her to be sympathetic and understanding. They knew very little about Trisomy 18, but she made the effort to get some information for the staff and I contributed what I had as well.*

It is important to be both sympathetic and informed. However, if you are unfamiliar with the baby's condition it is appropriate to seek information.

> *They made me think of what options I had open to me. It gave us the chance to decide on what level we wanted to care for our baby and what intervention we would allow. We decided that we wanted to give her every chance possible, but did not wish to 'prolong the inevitable'. In other words we wanted her to be comfortable and happy, but not on life support etc.*

Parents in this position may have to choose between spending a shorter time with the baby alive and in their arms and more time spent alive but in a neonatal intensive care unit (NICU). You can help them make this choice by arranging for them to visit the NICU and by discussing likely scenarios with them.

> *Tomorrow we'll be parents one way or another. Tomorrow will tell a thousand words. Please God let tomorrow be a happy day.*

For parents who have continued a pregnancy in the face of poor fetal diagnosis the birth day may well be the death day. Knowledge of this kind may be a source of great parental anxiety. Such anxiety may be alleviated if the parents know that all the health professionals involved in their care know the circumstances and are aware of their wishes without their having to state them over and over again. Therefore it is wise to discuss and document a birth plan that may include:

- the level of medication desired during labour and birth
- the amount of intervention preferred antepartum, intrapartum and postpartum, including views about Caesarean section in labour, and resuscitation efforts
- how the parents wish to spend their time in the immediate postpartum period
- what support people will be present and their role, e.g. someone to baptise the baby
- which ward area the parents wish to recover in or if they wish discharge as soon as possible
- postpartum pain relief.

THE ACTUAL BIRTH

As Grady and O'Leary (1993) say, it is important to make sure that parents understand the issues surrounding vaginal delivery and delivery by Caesarean section.

VAGINAL DELIVERY

Parents may:

- fear the baby may die before birth — most parents want as much time with the baby as possible
- fear that the act of pushing during vaginal birth may result in harm to or death of the baby
- like as much comfort as possible during labour — labour can be very frightening because it may mean the end of time with their baby

- want to birth the baby and have the baby on the mother's chest before any intervention
- not want the baby 'whisked' away — after the initial assessment many parents may want their baby with them for his whole lifetime if he is born alive
- like the option of having older siblings see their brother or sister alive

CAESAREAN BIRTH

Parents may:

- prefer the mother to remain awake in order to capture all of the baby's life, so an epidural/spinal anaesthetic is appropriate.
- wish to both be in the theatre and perhaps to have present a designated support person who can provide emotional support
- request that, after the birth, the partner go with the baby to NICU — the support person may then be a go-between to keep both parents informed of events

One family's story

Below is the story of one family's struggle after diagnosis of a chromosomal abnormality in their unborn baby. As you read, think about the following:

- whether informed choice was employed when the bad news was broken
- the prejudice the family encountered for not 'conforming'
- the ways the family coped and what you might suggest in a similar situation
- the half-truths/lies the mother was told and the possible motives for these
- the support the family received in hospital after the baby's birth
- the management and support the family received up to the time of death, including what feeding techniques the parents could have been taught to help in this situation.

At 18 weeks I had my first ultrasound — I thought it was so incredible — we could see the baby clearly and could see that little heart beating. The radiologist thought I was small for dates, so he suggested another scan in one week's time. My next scan seemed to last forever — they prodded and poked for about an hour. They couldn't find one of the joints of the little finger. I thought 'Who cares if it's missing part of its finger?' but they explained to me that this, along with the choroid plexus cysts, was a marker for Down syndrome. They suggested a specialist scan in the city (150 kilometres away) just to be sure.

At 20 weeks we travelled to the city. The night before the scan I felt my baby move for the very first time. It was a moment I had been waiting for and I was just so amazed at the feeling of life inside me.

We first had a meeting with a specialist who was all for termination even if it was Down syndrome. I found his attitude to lack any compassion whatsoever.

The scan found the 'missing' part of the baby's finger, but couldn't find another finger joint. It picked up the cysts, and thickening at the back of the neck, and a two-vessel umbilical cord. I was told that I had a 1:10 chance of having a baby with Down syndrome. I was offered an amniocentesis. I wasn't too sure about having this done, but didn't want to go back home and then wish I had done it, so we decided to have it done there and then. The results were to take about 2 weeks. We were both naturally upset and I think I cried all the way home. But the trip also gave us time to think and we both decided that we didn't care if our baby had Down syndrome, we'd love it no matter what!

Exactly 2 weeks to the day, I rang the specialist for the results. He came on the line and said 'The news is very bad. Your baby has Trisomy 18. It is fatal. All babies die. The baby won't even survive pregnancy, let alone birth. We advise you terminate immediately.' We went home believing we HAD to terminate this pregnancy. My own employer (also a medical professional) echoed the specialist's words and said 'You can go to the city and have the termination. Get it over now and get on with your life.'

I was a mess.

My husband came home. We cried, we talked and we cried some more. Then my baby started moving and kicking. Then and there we decided that while this baby was alive, we would do everything in our power to give it a chance. I rang the specialist back and asked what the sex of my baby was — he told me it was a little boy. We named him Peter and promised him we'd give him a chance at life.

I informed my doctor of my decision and I think he was horrified, but he said he'd do what he could. I think he was scared himself, he didn't know what to expect — Trisomy 18 is relatively rare.

The rest of my pregnancy was quite normal. Naturally we were both very anxious. I didn't sleep very much in those next 4 months. I'd lie down every afternoon, to savour the movements.

From the day I was diagnosed, I started to write a journal. I wrote down my thoughts and anxieties. I even wrote letters to Peter. That helped me cope.

Pressure came from all angles. My family were very, very supportive, but judgmental 'acquaintances' and doctors were anything but helpful. I'd hear back from lots of people thinking I was mad for continuing. The fact is I would have had to endure labour, whatever, so why not wait a little longer and give this little boy a chance? I felt that God would decide what was best and so, by leaving it in His hands, I wasn't really making any decisions.

A Caesarean section was planned because my doctor told me Peter was breech — I don't think he was. But I think by that stage my doctor was starting to be a little sympathetic. He might have felt that by not having to endure labour our baby might have a slight chance of being born alive.

The Caesarean was performed at 38 weeks. I had an epidural. I heard him cry as soon as he was lifted from me. It was music to my ears. He had a lot of trouble breathing but thanks to one doctor he was kept on oxygen and kept pink. I was taken back to my room where they presented me with Peter. We'd called a priest, who met us there, and Peter was baptised in my room. The paediatrician came in and told us it was 'very grave' and 'don't expect too much or too long'. His manner left a lot to be desired, as did his matter-of-fact attitude.

Peter did have a few more bouts of turning blue, but my husband would give him oxygen and 'pink' him up. In the early evening the baby breathed and stayed pink all on his own.

I found the hospital useless. There was one day when I didn't see a nurse from the first thing (when they brought him to me) till evening (when they took him away). A wonderful night nurse was on every night and she was the only one who tried to help him. She would sit for hours trying to feed him and then report back to me the amounts he'd taken. I will be forever grateful to this wonderful lady.

I was given false information on the amount of feed he should be having and so when I thought he was doing well, he was actually doing quite poorly.

On Day 5, I'd had enough. I decided I could do this better at home myself. We took him home and loved him.

The first night we were scared silly. He slept really well, we didn't!

At birth he weighed 4lb 6oz (1990gms). When I took him home he was only 3 lbs something.

So began the endless days of trying to get him to feed (poor sucking ability and tiring easily is a common problem for these precious babies). We did eye-dropper feeds, bottle feeds and even resorted to a 'possum bottle' from the vet. The possum bottle worked well for a while, but we needed to do more. I ended up with some midwives coming to the house and oral tube feeding him a couple of times a day with me bottle feeding the rest of the time. Then they had to come 4 times per day and I'd bottle feed at night. Then one night I just couldn't get him to feed at all. He'd gone from 9.00 p.m. the night before to 10.00 a.m. the next day without anything. A naso-gastric tube was inserted and we were able to feed him ourselves this way. His weight gains were immediate.

On a visit to the paediatrician at 6 weeks of age, we were told that he had a 'hole in the heart' (another common thing for this syndrome) and he told us that the increased food could put a strain on his heart. We really didn't have a choice though, he had to be fed, although some of the midwives who came to the house did suggest that we just dose him up on Panadol and 'let him go'!

His last weight gain was recorded at 1900 grams (just 90 short of his birth weight). We think he probably would have made it to his birth weight but ...

One night, 9 weeks and 2 days from his birth, we were just going to bed when he was sick. I changed him and wrapped him up and cuddled him to me in bed. I noticed his eyes were funny, I can't describe it, but certainly not normal. I called my husband and we pulled the tube from his nose, but he just stopped breathing. We did what we could to try to get him to breathe, but to no avail. It was very sudden, but peaceful and we were both there with him.

He was buried 3 days later.

We miss him terribly. He was all our hopes and dreams. I found it a nightmare for a long time. I had many really bad days. I returned to work 2 months later, to get out of the house.

I really needed to work then. But work had other ideas. They decided that I had brought all this grief upon myself by continuing with this pregnancy — they had no compassion. I worked a few months and then quit. I decided I didn't need people like that in my life any more.

We have learned who our friends are. There are many people I would not give the time of day to any more.

Almost 12 months after he passed away I found a support group called SOFT. It is a support group for families of Trisomy18, 13 and related disorders. I met many other people who are experiencing their T-18 babies, who have lost their T-18 babies and many more who are living day to day with their beautiful children. Some are even teenagers. That's right, one of the ladies I met has a son with T-18 who is 12 years of age.

> *Peter enriched our lives in many ways. We are both much stronger now and we know that we did the right thing. It would have been so easy to 'conform' and do what we were told to, but his little life meant a lot more to us than that.*

If, after a fetal diagnosis, parents elect to continue a pregnancy then they should expect from midwives and other health professionals the same nonjudgmental care and support that we give to parents whose baby is expected to be stillborn or die in the neonatal period (see Chapter 3).

If the baby is going to be born with obvious abnormalities which could be distressing to see, e.g. neural tube defects, then much of what is said under the heading, 'Meeting the baby' (see page 27) applies.

No regrets

> *My greatest comfort right now is that we never ran away from loving Eric. We were with him all the time, protecting him, defending him, and cherishing him. I believe that living with the pain of his dying is hard enough, but I am grateful that we have no guilt, or regrets. I think that the love we possess for our children can allow us to be fearless in loving them, even when we hurt so much.*

For this couple, and many like them, the four months of support and care during Eric's pregnancy afforded them the opportunity for anticipatory grieving. It was a time they valued and now treasure. They feel that if they had elected to terminate Eric's life they would have lived with guilt and regret as well as grief. As it is they have good memories and no regrets.

Organ donation?

Some parents, particularly those of anencephalic infants, may inquire about donating their baby's solid organs. Unfortunately this is not usually feasible because of legal reasons, notably the current definition of brain death (Peabody et al., 1989). Usually it is possible for the corneas to be 'harvested' after the baby's death.

FOSTERING?

It may be helpful for some couples to arrange for their baby to be fostered. This may give them the breathing space to decide what to do, as this family found:

> *We put our baby in temporary foster care for the first month of his life. We were devastated and needed to read up on Down syndrome and find out about it. We didn't want to become too attached to the baby in case we decided to give him up for adoption. Our 7-year old made the decision for us when he asked his father, 'Dad, if I break will you send me away? I'll help with the baby if he's broken.' Out of the mouths of babes! The truth in this statement is you can't predict the future for any of our children. And I think you would agree that if your child were hit by a car tomorrow and rendered handicapped, you would still love him or her, and do everything in your power to help him or her.*

Some parents feel they could not cope with raising a child with special needs, nor with terminating the pregnancy. For these couples, adoption may be a possible option. Exploring this option is best done with guidance from a genetic counsellor and/or another appropriate health professional such as an adoption caseworker or a social worker with experience in this area. Parents choosing this option may be faced with feelings of loss and uncertainty. As well, there will be grief associated with relinquishing their baby for adoption. (SAFDA, 1995: 18)

FOOT IN MOUTH

Here is a list of 'things that parents of children with any disability hate to hear from anyone' (including midwives) compiled by a mother of a baby with Down syndrome.

'I'm sorry', 'What a shame', 'How sad', 'Poor thing' . . . or any statement that conveys pity.

I came to dread any remarks that began with 'At least . . .'. I knew I would be hurt by whatever came next — 'At least your other child is normal.' (*Wow, that's real comforting.*)

Statements like:
'It could be worse.' No matter what the diagnosis at the time, nothing could be worse for the parent.
'They all look the same of course.' *No they don't!*
'How severely is he affected?' *He's not severe, he is my child.*

Any statement that puts blame on the parents. Don't say, 'It's a result of family problems' or 'It runs in families'. These statements imply that the parents are in some way responsible for their child's problems

'God only gives special children to special people.' Absolutely. The question is whether or not the parent chooses to accept the 'special' mantle and rise to the challenge presented by special children. God didn't choose me to parent a child with Down syndrome. But God did create a world where these things happen — sometimes to nice people, sometimes to not-so-nice people, sometimes to strong people, sometimes to weak people. What is important is what we do with what life hands us. The point is the process. Rather than being preordained, life is more like an improvisation. I choose to make it a dance.

Don't tell parents 'I couldn't do it.' 'I couldn't handle it.' 'You're a saint.' These statements imply that people with disabilities are so awful that only a saint would love and care for them. One mother says she always wants to reply, 'We have to handle what we're dealt, and maybe it isn't so easy for me to handle either.'

Don't imply that parents are brave. You are only brave if you have a choice. These parents have no choice.

REFERENCES

Clayton-Smith J, Farndon PA, McKeown C, Donnai D (1990): Examination of fetuses after induced abortion for fetal abnormality. *BMJ* 300 (6720) 3 Feb.:295–297.

Cooley WC et al. (1990): Reactions of mothers and medical professionals to a film about Down's Syndrome. *Am. J. Dis. Child* 144: 1112.

Grady G, O'Leary J (eds) (1993): *Heartbreak Pregnancies: Unfulfilled Promises.* Minneapolis: Abbott Northwestern Hospital.

Griffiths MJ et al. (1996): A false-positive diagnosis of Turner syndrome by amniocentesis. *Prenatal Diagnoses* 16 (5) May:463–466.

Julian-Reynier C et al. (1994): Fetal abnormalities detected by sonography in low-risk pregnancies: discrepancies between pre- and post-termination findings. *Fetal Diagn Ther* 9 (5) Sep.: 310–320.

Lette K (1996): *Mad Cows.* Pan MacMillan Australia: Sydney.

Merriam-Webster's Collegiate Dictionary, 10th edn (1998). Springfield: Merriam-Webster Inc.

Peabody JL, Emery JR, Ashwall S (1989): Experience with anencephalic infants as prospective organ donors. *The New England Journal of Medicine* August 321 (6): 344–350.

SAFDA (Support After Fetal Diagnosis of Abnormality) (1995): *Diagnosis of abnormality in an unborn baby . . . the impact, options and afterwards.* Sydney: NSW Genetics Education Program.

Waterson P, Richardson R (eds) (1998):*Appropriate Care for Women and Their Partners When Their Baby Dies,* 2nd edition. Sydney: SANDS, NSW.

INTERESTING RESEARCH ARTICLES

Dallaire L et al. (1995): Parental reaction and adaptability to the prenatal diagnosis of fetal defect or genetic disease leading to pregnancy interruption. *Prenat Diagn* 15 (3) Mar.: 249–259.

Drugan A et al. (1990): Determinants of parental decisions to abort for chromosome abnormalities. *Prenatal Diagnoses* 10 (8) Aug.:483–490.

Evans MI et al. (1993):The choices women make about prenatal diagnosis. *Fetal Diagn Ther* 8 Suppl 1, Apr.:70–80.

Evans MI et al. (1996): Parental decisions to terminate/continue following abnormal cytogenetic prenatal diagnosis: 'what' is still more important than 'when'. *Am J Med Genet* 61 (4) 2 Feb: 353–355.

Green R (1992): Letter to a genetic counsellor. *Journal of Genetic Counselling* 1:55–70.

Magyari PA et al. (1987): A supportive intervention protocol for couples terminating a pregnancy for genetic reasons. *Birth Defects Orig Artic Ser* 23 (6): 75–83.

Salvesen KA et al .(1997): Comparison of long-term psychological responses of women after pregnancy termination due to fetal anomalies and after perinatal loss. *Ultrasound Obstet Gynecol* 9 (2) Feb.: 80–85.

Sandelowski M, Jones LC (1996): Couples' evaluations of foreknowledge of fetal impairment. *Clin Nurs Res* 5 (1) Feb.: 81–96.

Sandelowski M, Jones LC (1996): Healing fictions: stories of choosing in the aftermath of the detection of fetal anomalies. *Soc Sci Med* 42 (3) Feb.: 353–361. Seller M et al. (1993): Grief and mid-trimester fetal loss. *Prenatal Diagnoses* 13 (5) May: 341–8.

Thomas J (1995): The effects on the family of miscarriage, termination for abnormality, stillbirth and neonatal death. *Child Care Health Dev* 21 (6) Nov.: 413–424.

White-Van Mourik MCA et al. (1992): The psychological sequelae of second trimester termination of pregnancy for fetal abnormality. *Prenatal Diagnoses* 12 (3): 189.

Zeanah CH et al. (1993): Do women grieve after terminating pregnancies because of fetal anomalies? A controlled investigation. *Obstet Gynecol* 82 (2) Aug.: 270–275.

RECOMMENDED READING

Boston S (1981): *Will, My Son — Life and Death of a Mongol Child.* London: Pluto Press.

Brill M (1988): *Keys to Parenting a Child with Down Syndrome.* New York: Barron's Educational Series.

Carson V (1990): *Beyond Prenatal Choice.* Omaha: Centering Corporation.

Creel MJ (1987): *A Little Death.* New York: Vantage Press.

Cunningham C (1982): *Down's Syndrome: An Introduction for Parents.* London: Souvenir Press

Davis D (1993): *Loving and Letting Go: For Parents Who Decide To Turn Away from Aggressive Medical Intervention for Their Critically Ill New-Borns.* Omaha: Centering Corporation.

Featherstone H (1980): *A Difference in the Family — Life with a Disabled Child*. London: Harper and Row.

Gryte M (1993): *Inner Healing after Abortion*. Omaha: Centering Corporation.

Hodge S (1995): *An Abortion for Love, Notes from a Friend: A Journal after a Genetic Termination*. Omaha: Centering Corporation.

Ilse S (no date): *Precious Lives, Painful Choices: A Prenatal Decision-making Guide* Maple Plain, MN: Wintergreen Press.

Johnson M, Johnson J (1988): *Difficult Decisions*. Omaha: Centering Corporation.

Katz Rothman B (1988): *The Tentative Pregnancy.* London: Pandora Press.

Lyon W, Minnick M (1993): *A Mother's Dilemma: A spiritual search for meaning following pregnancy interruption after prenatal diagnosis*. St Johns, MI: Pineapple Press.

Millard DM (1984): *Daily Living with a Handicapped Child*. London: Croom Helm.

Minnick M and Delp K with Ciotti M (1990): *A Time To Decide, A Time To Heal — for parents making difficult decisions about babies they love*. St Johns, MI: Pineapple Press.

Nicol M (1997): *Loss of a Baby.* Sydney: Harper Collins.

Panuthos C, Romeo C (1984): *Ended Beginnings: Healing Childbearing Losses*. South Hadley, MA: Bergin and Garvey Publisher's Inc.

Rich L (1991): *When Pregnancy Isn't Perfect*. New York: Dutton Books.

Scully T, Scully C (1989): *Making Medical Decisions*. New York: Simon and Schuster.

Segal M (1988): *In Time and With Love: Caring for the Special Needs Baby.* New York: Newmarket Press.

Simons R (1987): *After the Tears: Parents Talk About Raising a Child with a Disability*. Orlando: Harcourt Brace.

Spisak S, Pickett O (eds) (1993): *Children with Special Needs: A Resource Guide*. Arlington: National Center for Education in Maternal and Child Health.

CHAPTER 3

LATE PREGNANCY LOSS

I have a wish. Whenever I hold a dead baby, I wish that I will be able to find out the cause of its death and thereby prevent any further baby deaths and I wish that as I hold the baby it will wake up and I will be able to give it back to its parents.

(Pathologist, personal communication)

DEFINITION

The term 'late pregnancy loss' is defined variously. Used here it refers to any death which occurs from 20 weeks' gestation.

BREAKING BAD NEWS

> *I appreciated the fact she didn't lie to us or fob us off ... she simply and gently said 'I'm sorry, I can only find your heartbeat.'*

Bad news is best broken honestly and promptly. Most hospital protocol demands the medical officer be the bearer of bad news. However, you, as the midwife, are often in the unenviable position of being the first to suspect that something is wrong. If this happens then it is critical that you expedite the medical diagnosis.

The parents may be aware that there is something wrong. They may be coming to you to confirm an earlier diagnosis. On occasion, however, the baby's death will be sudden and unexpected.

Here is one midwife's account of sudden interuterine fetal death:

> In the early hours of one morning a couple presented to the hospital where I work. She was in labour with her first baby. They were very happy, although naturally a little anxious, about the impending birth.
>
> I took them into an examining room, chatting as I went. One of the questions I routinely ask is, 'Have you felt the baby moving this morning?' The answer was 'Yes.'
>
> I performed an abdominal palpation on her typically tight abdomen and the baby was easily palpated. I felt a fetal foot and commented to her that you could just about measure him for shoes! Even as these words left my mouth I wondered why the foot had not responded to my touch. I felt down the fetal back and applied a sonicaid. There was no sound, just absolute silence. I checked the machine. A feeling of dread hit me as I realised that the machine was on, the battery was charged and I was directly over the anterior shoulder. I should have been clearly hearing the fetal heart. Just in case, I shifted the sonicaid around a little in an attempt to hear something, anything, even placental noise, but there was no sound.
>
> I said to the parents 'I can't find your baby's heart beat. There may be something wrong. I'm going to get a doctor for an ultrasound.'
>
> The doctor confirmed my fear of fetal death in utero.
>
> On this occasion, when the parents left the hospital, I asked them how they thought I had handled the bad news. When I told them something might be wrong they had not believed me, in fact they thought I was an incompetent idiot. However, later, they had come to appreciate my actions.
>
> (Midwife, personal communication)

Tailor what you say to the situation and the individuals involved. All midwives regularly face instances where the fetal heart cannot be found easily and the reason may appear obvious, i.e. maternal size, fetal size or fetal mal-position. In these instances it is not constructive to create parental fear by suggesting to them that something is wrong. However, as soon as you are aware of a problem, the parents are entitled to an appropriate explanation.

Breaking bad news is one instance in which we need to consider professional judgment, skill, instinct and honesty.

How will they respond?

There are as many different responses to finding out bad news as there are people. Parents may be shocked into silence, they may scream, they may hit out at you, physically or in words, in their anger and disbelief. Regardless of response, they need a health professional who will be with them and stay with them.

Research has shown that nurses respond more easily to people who cry, sob or weep, but have greatest difficulty with those who withdraw into themselves (Wright, 1993). It is not easy to sit with someone who appears unaware of you, but it is important to be there for all people irrespective of their initial reactions. If either parent responds in anger — or they both do — it is important to stay with whoever is angry if at all possible. Remain calm yourself; try to defuse the anger by accepting it; encourage the couple to talk with you about why they are angry.

SUPPORT WHILE IN HOSPITAL AFTER BAD NEWS IS BROKEN

The midwife explained what she needed to do (i.e. contact the duty doctor) and got back to us promptly with his reply She offered us tea and coffee, ordered us breakfast and didn't bother us with any admission details or forms etc., and then made sure we were comfortable (e.g. when we expressed the need to get some sleep, she got a folding bed out for my husband). She was professional, but still showed human compassion. She included my husband in the conversation and answered his queries too.

You may be able to do some of the things in the following list.

- Provide a quiet room away from noise, especially the crying of other babies.
- Check that the parents have understood what has been said. Repeat any information that they may not have understood, especially any medical terms.
- Do not assume that parents know what is going on, especially if they are health professionals themselves. Bereaved health professionals may need to be told more rather than less.
- Provide explanations over and over again as needed. You are dealing with shocked people; don't expect too much from them. Be careful about how you 'explain' what has happened. One bereaved mother was concerned about a fever she had had prior to the baby's death. Her midwife replied before thinking, 'Yes, a high temperature can affect the baby . . . basically, it cooks them.' Mothers already carry enough guilt without our putting more on them.

- Provide written as well as spoken information. It is helpful for parents to have a ready reference to any information that is given to them.
- Give explanations of what will happen next.
- Sitting with the parents may be all that is required.
- Some couples will want immediate action, others will need time to absorb what has happened and assimilate what is likely to happen next. Avoid rushing parents unnecessarily into induction, delivery or any other procedure.
- Do not leave the parents alone for long periods. If you must leave provide an explanation and ensure someone else visits them while you cannot be there. They may experience absences as desertion:

  > *I was shut in a room and left alone for nearly 24 hours. No-one except my partner came to visit, no-one spoke to me. I felt isolated.*

- Allocate one person to act as co-ordinator for the family. This person will be their familiar face for the duration of their hospital stay and follow-up and will coordinate all aspects of care.

'I WANT A CAESAREAN'

It is not uncommon for parents to believe a Caesarean section under general anaesthetic will be 'easier'. This is especially so when the baby has died in utero and the mother faces enduring what might be considered a futile labour. The bereaved parents will need to understand the reasons why a vaginal birth is still advantageous.

Many obstetricians consider vaginal birth to be both physiologically and psychologically advantageous. In addition there are a number of reasons why Caesarean section is generally not advised in cases of late pregnancy loss:
- the uterus will be scarred and will therefore have an impact on subsequent pregnancies
- the woman has to recover from a major abdominal operation with the associated pain and increased recovery time
- the woman has a visible abdominal scar to remind her of her baby
- the physiological completion of the pregnancy in the normal way assists psychological closure.

However, it is also important to consider the woman's own opinions. One bereaved parent I met requested a Caesarean and after quizzing her carefully, the obstetrician did proceed with the surgery. This woman's rationale was convincing: she had endured a difficult forceps delivery with her first baby and a subsequent long recovery after the birth. Her request was considered valid as she felt that her recovery after the Caesarean section was likely to be quicker and less physically painful than the forceps birth.

A WORD ABOUT EMERGENCIES

Once the cord prolapsed I had to get up onto the bed in a head down, tail in the air position and my contractions were coming thick and strong. I had people all around me doing things to me and I had a doctor with her arm in me holding the baby's head off the cord and the amount of pain I felt was just incredible and I just felt like the medical staff forgot I was a person. It was an emergency and they were trying to save the baby's life and look after me but I felt like a piece of meat on that table just being violated.

(From the video, *A Part of You Dies*)

It is very important during an emergency to maintain the lines of communication and to remember that the parents are usually very afraid and do not know what is going on.

CLINICAL MANAGEMENT

(*expected vaginal stillbirth*)

AS IF THE BABY WERE ALIVE

> The doctor told us to treat her like a newborn baby and that was really good advice.
>
> (From the video, *A Part of You Dies*)

This is really good advice. When caring for bereaved families, always ask yourself 'What would I do if this baby were alive?'

CONTINUITY OF MIDWIFE

Bereaved parents may be more likely to become confused. They will not remember easily much of what is said or done to them. It is therefore important, as far as possible, to reduce the number of people responsible for the care of the family. A small team will be better able to monitor what happens.

PAIN RELIEF

A woman who is shocked and numb is unlikely to be able to make a clear decision. She may accept whatever you suggest to her. Medical staff commonly believe that women experiencing vaginal stillbirth will want a pain-free labour. However, this may not be the case.

> *When my baby was found to be dead, I felt like the only thing I had left was a normal vaginal delivery. I didn't want the epidural or the trappings of the epidural like the drip and the sore back. I wanted to feel everything that was happening to me.*

Offer strong pain relief with caution. I have heard many women say that they do not have a clear memory of their baby's birth. The strong pain relief they were given clouded their perceptions. They felt 'out of it' at the birth and when they 'came round' they felt unable to ask for their baby.

> *I used a shower to help in labour. For the first few weeks at home, every time I had a shower I relived the pain of labour.*

Avoid routinely offering baths and showers as pain relief in case regular ablutions become associated with distressing flashbacks. If the woman prefers this kind of pain relief it may be wise to warn her about possible consequences of this choice.

Women who elect not to have an epidural may be offered TENS (transcutaneous electrical nerve stimulation) or nitrous oxide. Both are short-acting and effective.

MANAGEMENT OF THE BIRTH

The worst part of my labour experience was being able to hear a baby's heartbeat on the fetal heart monitor in the room nextdoor.

Consider the impact of where the couple are situated in the delivery suite and try to minimise distress by turning monitors down or off. If there is a choice, place bereaved families in a room which is quiet and away from the 'action'.

WHAT WILL THE BABY LOOK LIKE?

Many parents will ask you what the baby will look like. It can be very difficult for midwives to predict, especially if the time since death is uncertain. Degree of maceration will vary, as will colour of the baby's skin. Some may be red, especially if pre-term; others may be white, especially if the baby has bled, e.g. vasa praevia. It is difficult, if not impossible, to predict accurately what the baby will look like.

If a baby is to be born alive, you do not tell the parents that he is likely to be pink with blue hands and feet, covered with vernix mixed with maternal blood and maybe even a green or yellow colour from meconium staining! These things are unimportant and generally go unnoticed because the parents want to meet their baby.

Bereaved parents also want to meet their baby. I believe that when bereaved parents ask you what their baby will look like their question is based more on their fear of the unknown than their curiosity about their baby's likely appearance. Therefore say something like 'I don't know what he will look like but he is your precious baby. He will be warm from your body and I will deliver him onto your tummy so you can see him straight away.'

It is becoming increasingly common to deliver a living baby straight onto the mother's abdomen to encourage 'bonding' and skin-to-skin contact. Why would you not do this just because you know the baby is dead? The baby is still the parents' longed-for, much-wanted baby.

Parents will be guided by what you do and say. If you act 'naturally' then they are much more likely to accept your actions as usual and act 'naturally' too.

If it is known that the baby has been dead for several days then it is important to prepare parents to expect some maceration. If the baby is expected to be macerated, contact can still occur. This situation does, however, demand an explanation from you of the baby's likely appearance and probable causes of the deterioration.

WHAT IF THEY REALLY DON'T WANT TO SEE THEIR BABY?

> *The hospital took pictures for us, and my husband and I have never seen them. They are still at the hospital, ready for us when we are ready for them.*

There will be parents who tell you they don't want to see their baby; who, despite your best endeavours, refuse to see and cuddle their baby. The midwife's role as advocate is paramount here. Two things need to be done.
- the parents need to be gently but firmly encouraged to change their minds.
- the midwife needs to go ahead and create mementoes anyway, telling the parents that they have been collected and will be kept safe until they are ready for them.

CHANGING THEIR MIND

Fear may well be the driving force in parents deciding not to see the baby, particularly if there is abnormality or maceration involved. Midwives need to acknowledge the parents' fear but work through it to produce an acceptance of the baby as a person, entitled to acknowledgement irrespective of how he looks.

One tactic which usually does not work is quoting research or statistics. It is not helpful for bereaved parents to learn that their grief will be easier or less complicated if they see their baby, nor that their grief will be facilitated by seeing and holding their dead infant (Moscarello, 1989). Neither will they benefit from knowing that most bereaved parents regret not seeing their baby but few regret they did. It is we midwives who must work from these facts, encouraging parents gently to change their mind.

Say things like 'He is your beautiful baby, you won't be sorry you saw him'; 'It will be OK, we'll just take it slowly'; 'He has your nose'; 'He has his father's big feet.' Use language like 'Other parents have found it beneficial to . . .' rather than 'Research shows that . . .'

If parents do not change their mind while they are still under your care, they need to know that there will be opportunities for them to change their mind and that you intend to gather mementoes and keep them in case they request them later.

It may be that the parents are reluctant to hold their baby. If you think this is the case, you hold the baby because if you are reluctant to hold their baby they will be too. Wrap the baby in a warm blanket. Describe the baby, noticing 'good' features — 'perfect' little hands, 'sweet' little nose. Use the baby's name and talk to the baby using his name. Approach the parents gradually, watching out for body language that indicates whether your approach is being welcomed or rejected. Talk to the baby and fondle him more if you are getting negative messages.

Be aware of your facial expression. To allow horror to show may inhibit parents' natural desire to see and cuddle their baby. Take the parents' hands and place them over yours if they still appear afraid

GOING BEHIND THEIR BACKS

If parents do not change their mind and decide to see their baby then it is of crucial importance that all mementoes are still taken. In some ways it is even more important, because it is extremely likely that they will change their mind.

It is best to have someone hold the baby when photos are taken. It may be the midwife who delivered the baby but ideally it should be a member of the family. The mother's partner may be amenable to being photographed with the baby. Many men fall naturally into what can be called a 'loving, protective role', meaning they will attempt to protect their spouse from any further possibility of hurt or harm (see Appendix 2). In fact the male may be the one who is not allowing his spouse to cuddle the baby, in the misguided attempt to protect her from having to 'endure' contact with the baby whilst she is distressed. Midwives may be able to use this natural 'protective' response to encourage the male to have photos taken with the baby. Once the male has had contact with his baby he may decide it is okay after all and he may then be influential in helping his spouse to meet their baby too.

If the partner is unwilling then you may discreetly ask the grandparents. These people often feel helpless when their grandchild dies and may respond well to your suggestion that they will be helping their child by seeing and cuddling and being photographed with their grandchild. Here is an example of what happened when a funeral director was thoughtful enough to use a grandparent to go behind a mother's back:

> *When our baby was in the hospital he wore a plain blue jumpsuit. We did not want him to be buried in it, preferring to buy something new and smart and warm. The jumpsuit then became superfluous.*
>
> *When we went to the funeral parlour to see our baby for the last time one of the first things the attending funeral director said was 'Here is his jumpsuit' and she offered me a plain, brown paper bag. I replied, 'No thanks', left the jumpsuit on a nearby table and went on in to see our baby and cuddle him for the last time. Unbeknown to me the undertaker found the jumpsuit after we had left and put it with the things to be taken to the funeral. At the funeral she gave it to my mother saying, 'Keep this for your daughter, she will ask for it one day.'*
>
> *Needless to say, a week or so after the funeral I realised that I needed to have that jumpsuit as a memento. Our baby had worn the suit and it carried his scent. I made many calls to both the funeral parlour and the social worker at the hospital*

trying to find out what had happened to it, but no-one knew. I resigned myself to the fact that it had been discarded.

Many weeks later I complained about this apparent lack of caring to my mother and she said 'Oh I wouldn't be too harsh on them, I have it!' I simply could not believe that my mother had something that had become so precious to me but which I thought was lost forever. When she gave it to me, it was like getting a little bit of my baby back.

I am so grateful that when that funeral director heard 'No' she knew I didn't mean no for ever just no for now.

WHICH WARD?

What do you do with a person whose baby has been stillborn and who needs hospital care for a few days postpartum? Leaving her in the labour ward exposes her to the sights and sounds of happy pregnant women having live healthy babies. Moving her to a postnatal ward means continued bombardment with the noise of crying babies. Caring for such couples on a gynaecology ward may seem the kindest option but what about the staff? Are they qualified to care for postnatal women? And what about the baby rooming in? All these options are fraught with difficulty. Certainly the couple themselves need to be involved in the decision.

Another option may be for the hospital to provide a quiet room away from the hubbub of the hospital where parents, particularly fathers, can come and go with their baby and other children, neither disturbing others with living babies nor having those with living babies disturbing them. I know of a hospital where the local SANDS organisation has set up a room large enough for several family members, with a double bed, a lounge suite, comfortable chairs, a kitchenette with tea- and coffee-making facilities, tissues, a phone and a call bell, with attractive decor and a cot for the baby. This room is located near a stairwell at the back of a postnatal ward. Parents can come and go as they please, taking their baby outside if they wish, but still having full access to nursing staff and nursing care. This arrangement is ideal. Your hospital may be able to emulate some if not all of this set-up. Such a room can be part of a maternity unit's design. It may be used not only for dying babies but also for parents of acutely/critically ill babies who may wish to stay the night close to their baby. One woman had this experience at a country hospital:

Initially we were in a room in the maternity section but when the ultrasound confirmed our baby had died . . . we were offered the use of a 'family unit' at the other end of the hospital. It is a suite of rooms usually reserved for palliative care patients and people in situations like ours. It's a wing of the hospital where a few rooms at one end are used for day-surgery patients twice a week and it also has a few offices in it. So it is isolated and very private and suited our needs extremely well! It was great being out of the maternity wing and not having to worry about bumping into other mothers or hearing their babies cry.

The unit we used had its own private bathroom, 2 bedrooms and a lounge room so other family members could visit or sleep overnight. One bedroom was a typical hospital room and the other contained a sofa bed and coffee table. This was the room my husband slept in. It meant he was close by, but an adjoining door could be closed so the comings and goings of the midwives during the night didn't disturb him. There was plenty of space for our 2 girls to play and watch TV in the lounge room and they and my parents were allowed to visit us freely at any time.

Many women find it comforting to have their partner accommodated with them. This person needs access to food and ablution facilities.

TIME ALONE

When the paediatrician had told us that Helen had gone, the midwives, who were mostly crying themselves, asked us if we wanted some time on our own with Helen. We said we did and they left us holding her. They told us just to call when we were ready for anyone to bath Helen or for them to sort me out — I needed stitches. Having those first few minutes alone, just the three of us, helped us cope with the initial shock, anger and grief. It was good to be private even though there were so many things that needed doing. We started taking pictures of her at that point. I suppose we had her for about 10 minutes or so.

ROOM-IN

It is ideal to room the baby in. Parents then have the option to look at or cuddle the baby or leave the baby in the cot. If the parents do not want their baby in their room, make provision for the baby to be kept in the ward rather than the morgue, especially as the morgue is often quite distant from the maternity unit. Some hospitals have a special small refrigerator in the delivery room area. The baby may be kept in such a refrigerator overnight or at other times if the parents wish some time away from the baby. If the baby is placed in a refrigerator it may be helpful to rub small amounts of cold cream into the skin (if the skin is intact) — this may help to preserve it. It is also important not to wrap baby too tightly and to avoid bumps and lumps in the wraps as these can permanently indent the baby's skin. If the baby has spent time in the refrigerator then it is important to use a warm wrap when returning the baby to the parents for a cuddle.

ANCILLARY STAFF

The hospital put a single rose on the outside of my door. This let all staff know that I had just experienced a loss so that they would know before entering my room.

In order to minimise distress to the newly bereaved parents all staff from midwife through to physiotherapist, hospital photographer, volunteers and cleaner need to be made aware that the couple in the room have lost a baby. One of the easiest ways of effecting this is to have some kind of symbol on the door inviting visitors to check with the nursing staff before entering the room. This alerts staff without placing pressure on anyone to maintain vigilance outside the door. This also makes it much less likely that someone will barge in without being aware of the situation. A discussion needs to occur prior to the symbol's use so the parents are aware of the reasons why it is used and what its use will attempt to achieve. It is very important to point out that some people may still not see the sign so it will minimise, rather than eliminate, such situations.

CLINICAL MANAGEMENT

(*neonatal death*)

RESUSCITATION

If attempts are made to resuscitate the baby, it is very important that the parents are present, but they will need debriefing afterwards. It is vital, however, not to say anything to the parents unless you are sure, or reasonably sure, because what you say can lead to distress, as this mother found:

> *While the paediatric team were trying to resuscitate Helen, one midwife, by my head, kept telling me everything was going to be okay. As time went on, I knew we had lost her and I just wanted the midwife to go away.*

NEONATAL INTENSIVE CARE UNIT (NICU)

When a baby requires admission to a NICU the parents are likely to need much reassurance and sensitivity to their needs, especially if the NICU is situated in another hospital.

After the birth, intensive care technology can have two contradictory effects on parents. There is the reassurance that everything possible is being done to treat their baby, but on the other hand the complexity of technology imposes a barrier between parents and baby (Thearle and Gregory, 1992).

> I was able to touch him but I had expected to be able to hold him and to be told that to hold him would de-stabilise him was . . . I don't know I just felt stunned. I felt like this is my baby. Whose baby is it? Surely a mother can hold her baby.
>
> Anyway I begged the doctor and was permitted to hold him for 10 minutes and that felt really good and seemed to calm me down just being able to hold him. I wish that someone had simply guided me by saying 'your baby really needs you and needs to be touched by you and it's really important that you are a part of his care. He knows you are here. He can't respond to that but he knows'
>
> (From the video, *A Part of You Dies*)

Prior to admission or transfer to a NICU the parents need:
- information about the baby's condition and reasons for intensive care
- an opportunity to a least touch but ideally to hold their baby
- an introduction to the staff who will be caring for the baby during inter-hospital transfer
- an instant photo if one or other of them cannot immediately accompany the baby
- an opportunity to ask questions
- information about how their baby may look, including likely tubes, as well as likely procedures, care etc.

SPENDING TIME WITH THE BABY

> When I found out he was going to die I didn't want to look at him any more. I didn't want to nurse him. They offered me but I said 'no thanks'. Now when I look back I know it was my way of protecting myself. I thought, 'If I don't look at him, don't nurse him, don't cuddle him I won't love him therefore it won't hurt.' I realise now that that wasn't the case. Thankfully, one of the sisters convinced me to have a cuddle and I never put him down after that.
>
> (From the video, *A Part of You Dies*)

- It is helpful to encourage parents to have physical contact with their baby.
- It is important to familiarise the parents with the various medical equipment in use around their baby, especially alarms and what they mean, as well as routine procedures and care their baby is receiving.
- It is vital to tell the parents that they are a crucial part of their baby's care.

CARING FOR THE BABY

If it is at all possible, many parents appreciate the chance to care for their baby. Simple procedures may be performed under staff guidance. Encourage the parents to engage in parenting activities such as bathing, washing, changing and dressing. Such opportunities may become precious memories after their baby's death.

Feeding may also be encouraged if it is feasible. If it is known that the baby will die, breastfeeding may still be desirable. Many bereaved mothers treasure their memories of breastfeeding their dying baby.

WITHDRAWING LIFE SUPPORT

It may be important for some parents to discuss withdrawal of life support with other members of their family and friends.

> We had a meeting with the doctor to decide whether to remove our baby from the life support and at that meeting we decided that that was the best thing to do at the time because his condition was deteriorating rapidly. The doctor felt he would probably live a few days to a few weeks and we had decided that we would take him home and care for him at home.
>
> There was a sense of relief and a feeling of at last I'll be able to mother my child in some form for a very short while. But when the equipment was removed he died very quickly and neither my husband nor I were there. I will always regret that the doctor didn't think 'I'm not God, I don't know when this child will die, really. Maybe we can just leave the child on for a while longer while the parents rest so they can be there in case he dies.'
>
> For me I felt like I never performed a single act of caring for my baby and to have nursed him out of this life would have been the one very special thing I could have done for him.
>
> (From the video, *A Part of You Dies*)

If the decision is made to remove the baby from life support, parents need to be given the option as to whether to be present or not. Most parents will choose to nurse their baby 'out of this life' but will need to be supported during this time. Most require an explanation of how the baby will be and what he will look like. Many will need to be reassured that the baby will not struggle for breath. Most parents will not have seen a person die before, let alone a baby, and may have a 'Hollywood' image of what dying is like. The idea of being with their baby when the baby dies is therefore likely to be very frightening for parents.

> *If we only had time to prepare and could do it all over again. If only we realised the finality of what we were facing and if only we weren't in emotional shock and a bit of denial at a time we should have been clearheaded. I'll always regret that I never kissed him goodbye. To this day it has always bothered me that he never knew a mother's kiss.*

Parents always need to know:

- how the decision to withdraw treatment was arrived at, i.e. what happened to bring things to this point
- how long their child is expected to live and the advantages versus the disadvantages of available treatment
- what is likely to happen if treatment is continued, including how long the baby's life is likely to go on
- what is actually wrong in plain language, e.g. 'stiff lungs' rather than 'HMD' (hyaline membrane disease)
- what to expect, i.e. how their child will deteriorate and die, including whether there will be pain and how this will be dealt with
- how to plan for the death, i.e. who will be there, where, and when
- what options there are for support, e.g. good friend, social worker, chaplain etc.
- that their baby will be cared for by as few staff as possible
- what skills will be needed to care for their baby if they do decide to take him home, e.g. tube feeding, wound care, maintaining airway, oxygen therapy etc.

Midwives need to be aware of religious rites but should not attempt to perform any unless specifically asked by the parents and only when there is no time to call an appropriate minister/priest.

As midwives we also need to be aware of our own attitudes towards withdrawing treatment for any given baby.

> We're sensitive to the fact that sometimes the nursing staff may not agree with our decisions. It is very important, and has now become part of our normal process, to have group meetings and discussions about this, and we are certainly very sensitive to staff who disagree with decisions, and where possible, try and help them through that. Still, I think, it is parents that have the final say, and should be involved in the final decision making, but if staff are in disagreement with decisions, we have to help them through that process as well. (McPhee, 1995)

WHERE

Some parents may like to choose where their baby dies. This may or may not be in the NICU. It is best to try to be flexible and to respect the parents' choice if it is at all possible.

Home

> We brought him home in the car, which I found extremely difficult — I was
> frightened he was going to die on the way home. We got to spend a lot of time,
> we were able to do things with him — cuddle him, bath him, take him for
> walks, all the things you do with babies. It was wonderful.
>
> (From the video, *A Part of You Dies*)

Some parents may be afraid to take their baby home, but once they are
home may find the whole experience is very worthwhile. Inform the
parents that the hospital is still available to support them when their baby
dies. If the parents find they cannot cope with the dying baby's care at
home then they should feel welcome to return to hospital.

Hospital

Provision of a room within the hospital or a private area within the hospital
grounds may be appropriate. If the parents elect to take the baby into the
hospital grounds or to an outside park then a pram may be supplied.

> We actually have a room that is quite separate from the nursery, that doesn't
> look into the nursery, to be available for this process. In fact, the room is fully
> equipped to have the child in there still on the ventilator, providing intensive
> care, and the process of removal of the tube can happen with the parents,
> with privacy. (McPhee, 1995)

THE DYING

> *Someone is dying in your arms and you can't stop it!*

It is very important for midwives to help parents plan and own their
baby's dying to minimise regrets and to make the experience as 'good' as
it can be given the circumstances.

Parenting the dying baby

It is vital, once the decision is made to remove life support, that the parents
are not rushed. The story below is an example of the kind of care that can
be offered:

> *Our baby's nurse took off all his monitors and let us give him*
> *a bath. I had asked for his footprints, so we did that then (we*
> *already had a lock of hair). Mike and I left the room for a few*

minutes while the nurse took out his tubes. She also dressed him in a jumpsuit and wrapped him in a blanket. When we came back, I sat in a rocking chair and they put our baby in my arms. I got to hold my son for the first time. Through all the tears and the incredible pain, I got great pleasure out of holding him. He still had the breathing tube in. They draped the tubes over my shoulder and tied them to the chair. The ventilator was still on and he had morphine for pain, but all the other tubes and wires were gone. I just held him close, feeling his softness and warmth, and smelling his sweet baby smell. He was pretty sedated, but I'm sure he could hear me. I talked to him through my tears, telling him how much I loved him. I kissed him and snuggled as much as possible.

After about an hour, we called the doctors over and told them they could removed his life support. One of the doctors removed the tape from our baby's mouth and took the tube out of his throat. I was still holding him as he died in my arms. Mike held him then for a few minutes and I held him again. We stayed there for about 45 more minutes, just crying, holding our son, talking to him, and loving him.

HOW MIDWIVES CAN HELP PARENTS CARE FOR THEIR DYING BABY

Most bereaved parents value the memories they have of the time they spent with their dead or dying baby. It is important to provide parenting activities whether the baby is alive or dead. Some or all of these suggestions may be appropriate.

- Give the parents privacy. Provide opportunities for the parents to leave the room if they wish. Assist parents but leave them some privacy too.

- Encourage parents to talk to their baby. If baby is named it is ideal to use the baby's name and encourage parents to do the same. Invite them to tell their baby what they would like him to know. Ask them, 'What would you like to tell him? If he could talk what would you like him to tell you?' Write down this conversation, keep a copy and put the other aside to place in the coffin.

• Invite the parents to watch someone bath their baby or, ideally, help them bath the baby themselves. Create a scent memory at this stage by placing scented water in the bath or using a scented baby powder after the bath — rose is nice but have a range available.

• Suggest parents play music, sing lullabies, change nappies, dress/undress their baby or take the baby for a walk outside in a pram.

• Encourage significant others (siblings, grandparents) to share and have contact with the baby and the parents. If siblings are involved it may be appropriate for them to give their dying sibling a present and 'receive' one from him. Encourage siblings to write a letter or draw a picture for their baby

• Even if parents do not wish to take their baby home, encourage them to carry the baby out of the hospital as they would have if he were alive.

I remember the hardest thing of the whole period was when we left the hospital. When we were finally left alone in the room with the baby, we were going to go but for God knows what reason we weren't going to take him with us. We were going to leave him behind at the hospital. Neither of us could do it. We didn't want to put him down and say, 'Bye bye' and walk out. That was so hard that after that everything else seemed easier because it was honestly like ripping my arm off to put him down in the cot and walk out of the room.

(From the video, *A Part of You Dies*)

If you are unsure about 'allowing' any of these things to happen ask yourself two questions 'Would I allow it if the baby was alive?' and 'What is the worst thing that could happen if they did it?'

CARING FOR THE PARENTS

> I asked for a sleeping tablet, which didn't work. I must have walked past the nurses' station 20 times that night going out, having a cigarette, coming back, trying to go to sleep, and they would just look at me and nobody ever said a word. I was very angry that nobody gave me the choice. I mean I would have liked someone to say 'Would you like some company?' rather than just presuming that I wanted to be on my own, because I didn't. I didn't even necessarily want to talk about the baby. I just wanted somebody to be there with me, just to have someone near me.
>
> (From the video, *A Part of You Dies*)

If one or both of the parents are still in your care, particularly after the baby has died, they may feel that they need some adult contact or conversation to relieve the tension they are feeling. Best practice may include giving them some company or an outlet for conversation. It is not necessarily important to talk about the baby. It may be best to let the parents lead the conversation.

AUTOPSY

Timing of the request for autopsy needs to be sensitive. Some bereaved parents have been especially distressed when the request for the autopsy has preceded their baby's death! If the autopsy is required legally then the parents need a clear explanation of the reasons for this. Their options for partial autopsy must also be fully explained. If the autopsy is not legally required then parents need to be fully aware that the autopsy cannot be performed without their written consent.

> *I rang the funeral parlour and asked if I could go and have another cuddle of my baby. The lady there said 'No, dear, you see the baby would have had her little operation.' I said that I hadn't consented to an autopsy. The lady replied 'But, dear, they all have their little operations before they come here!' I literally flew down to the funeral parlour and virtually tore my baby's clothes off in order to satisfy myself that she hadn't had the autopsy without my consent. It was most distressing.*

If the parents elect to have an autopsy, most parenting opportunities need to occur prior to the autopsy taking place. If the baby is very small or macerated, repair after autopsy may be difficult or even impossible.

These parents need to be aware that they may not be able to hold their smaller baby after the autopsy. Bigger babies are usually placed in a body suit and dressed prior to the parents seeing them again.

Autopsy may provide parents with information about what went wrong and may give guidelines about possible investigations, as happened in this case:

> *I am glad he had an autopsy. I am glad because my most pressing questions were not 'Why?' but rather 'How?' I wanted to know what exactly had gone wrong, and put aside any question of fault. After the autopsy, we learned that he had died from a genetic disorder (which caused his defects) and there was absolutely nothing we could have done to prevent it (and by nature, nothing we did to cause it). That was most reassuring.*

Before they give permission for an autopsy parents must be made aware that, generally, autopsy is required by law only if the medical officer cannot determine the cause of a neonatal death. If the cause of death is known there can be an autopsy to confirm it, but it is the parents' choice. There may be objections to autopsy on religious grounds (see Appendix 5). It is important for parents to understand:
- why the autopsy is requested
- when and where it will be done
- what happens during the autopsy
- that the baby's arms, legs and face are generally not touched.

Parents need to be aware that the post-mortem may not show conclusively their baby's cause of death, although it may rule out some suspected causes of death. They also need to know when they will get the results and that the results will be explained to them. Many parents appreciate the opportunity to discuss the findings of the autopsy with the pathologist who performed the examination.

Alternatives

> *He had a full-body x-ray and ultrasound as well as blood and chromosome testing on the placenta. None of these showed any abnormality so we decided not to go ahead with the full autopsy as we felt sure that they wouldn't be able to shed any more light on the reason for his death.*

Some parents may be reluctant for a full autopsy but may consent to noninvasive alternatives. Information gained from these investigations can also be very helpful in determining the cause of the baby's death.

Partial autopsy

Partial autopsy examines only those organs thought to be the likely cause of death.

> *Our son died of a cardiac abnormality. We therefore gave permission for a partial autopsy to look at the heart and lungs only. We knew there was nothing else wrong with him and didn't want to put ourselves through another operation, even one after his death.*

The placenta is an important part of the autopsy as its tissue is the same as the baby's. The placenta should be labelled and sent to the histopathology laboratory. It must be sent fresh (no preservatives) and if there is likely to be a delay of more than 12 hours before it is examined, it must be refrigerated. Clearly label twin placentas 'Twin 1' and 'Twin 2'.

Pathology tests

Pathology tests usually contribute to understanding the cause of the baby's death. Blood tests will vary from centre to centre but these are most usual:

Cord blood: Fetal blood often cannot be obtained at autopsy but it may be possible to take cord blood at delivery. A complete blood picture, group, Rh factor and antibody level, direct Coombs', and chromosome studies will all be performed if possible.

Maternal blood: The mother's blood should be taken and tested for Kleihauer (fetal blood) and serology, e.g. toxoplasmosis. If the mother is Rh negative, an indirect Coombs' test should also be included.

REASONS FOR MEMORY CREATION

Why is such emphasis placed on memory creation and how do we help parents do this?

There are many milestones in our lifetime when photos are usually taken — first smile, first step, first day at kindergarten, first day at school etc. A photo keeps the image of such milestones before us. In much the same way, taking photos of a baby who dies keeps the baby's image before the parents, affirming to them that their baby was real. Photographs confirm the baby's existence. Placing a photo or other memento of the baby in the family home allows the baby a place in the family. Most families have on display photos of their living children, parents, or grandparents. Even when family members die, most bereaved people do not remove photos because the person remains a part of the family, albeit absent. It is very important for many bereaved families to have their dead baby recognised as an absent member of the family. Further, the presence of a photo or other memento in the family home may provide an opportunity to share the baby with others.

Bereaved parents need to have something tangible of their baby. This is important, both in the early days of grief and further down the track. Parents need to have a focus for release of their sorrow and a concrete memento to assist them to remember their baby.

A MOST IMPORTANT PICTURE

One comment I hear more than any other from bereaved parents is *'I wish I had more photos.'* It is absolutely crucial that photos are taken and plenty of them, with as many different cameras and photographers as possible, to maximise the number of photos the bereaved parents have.

When?

> *Before they bathed him they took a couple of Polaroid (instant) photos of him so we had something immediate.*

Contact and photo opportunities are best within a few hours of stillbirth or neonatal death whilst the baby is still warm and minimal post-mortem changes have taken place.

What?

Take photos with as 'good' a camera as possible and with more than one camera (in case the film or camera is faulty). Ensure there is film in the camera!

It is important to take photos with a camera that produces an instant photo, especially if there are children involved. It is ideal to show children a photo before they see their sibling. 'Instant' cameras have their disadvantages — they do not usually produce a high-quality photo and the photos fade over time. It is recommended that such photos be copied by a professional photographer so that a more permanent photo is produced. Tell parents to take only one photo at a time or one film at a time to be processed rather than risk all of them being lost.

Many hospitals have professional photographers who visit on a regular basis to take photos of living infants. Most are willing, for the usual fee, to take photos of a dead or dying infant and the resulting photographs should be close-ups of high quality.

Most hospitals have clinical photographers who also have good-quality cameras. They may also be willing, perhaps for a fee, to take a series of photos of the infant.

'Disposable' cameras are now held in stock by many hospitals to give to parents to take photos to be processed at their expense if and when they desire.

If the parents have consented to a post-mortem many pathologists take photographs to give to parents. Such photos are taken prior to autopsy and are usually of high quality.

How?

Imagine the baby is alive and take photos with this in mind.
- Take as many photos as possible with as many people as possible in as many different angles/positions as possible, inside and outside and at different times of the day to maximise the chances of some good photos.
- Take group shots as triangles rather than in a straight line. A triangle has a warmer feel.

- Include at least one photo of the baby in the room where he was born.
- When taking photos of family members, wait a few moments for the person to start interacting with the baby and the photo will be more meaningful. Ask the person to look at the baby rather than at the camera. People will smile more naturally at the baby than at the camera.
- Take as many different aspects of the baby as possible, both naked and clothed. Memories fade and many parents forget they saw their baby naked at all. Some feel that they can't remember seeing the gender of their baby:

> *Unfortunately, I can't tell you what his body looked like, because we never undressed him, something I will regret until the day I die. Odd as it sounds, we didn't want to disturb him.*

- Use natural light if possible as flash light is harsh.
- Be aware of the baby's colour and the colour of the surround. A very pale baby will get lost in the picture if dressed in white and laid on white. A very red baby will clash horribly with surgical green and this colour combination is best avoided!
- Even imperfect babies have a perfect feature — maybe the feet, an ear or a hand. Take close-up photos of the perfect feature.
- Wrap the baby loosely — a tightly wrapped baby may give an Egyptian 'mummy' appearance.
- Arrange the baby to look as much like a sleeping baby as possible. Placing the baby on his side may be a way of achieving this.
- Dress the baby, place an appropriate toy of an appropriate size with the baby and take the time to arrange the baby's fingers so that it appears to be holding the toy.
- The cot or baby basket size needs to be in keeping with the size of the baby. A doll's basket or cut-down baby rugs may be required so parents can focus on their baby.

What else?

If photos are refused it is absolutely crucial they are taken anyway, unless the objection is on religious or cultural grounds.

Encourage the parents to compile a photo/memory album when they are ready. Prepare them for the fact that the appearance of this album may change several times as they feel comfortable about adding or creating more mementoes.

Initially I just had photos but over time I added his birth certificate, baptism certificate, cuttings from the newspaper, funeral order of service etc. When we redecorated his room for the new baby I even put into the album some of the wallpaper border we had chosen for him.

- Photos can also become portraits at the hands of a skilled artist. Portraits can be done in colour pastel or charcoal. The artist can take some artistic licence and omit discoloration or peeling skin to reproduce the likeness of the baby as he would have appeared if circumstances had been different. It is also possible to sketch the entire family together and thereby create a family 'shot'. Another alternative is to have all children from one family sketched as babies on the one portrait.
- Photos may be reduced in size and placed in a locket or made into a key ring.
- Consider using video to record events around the birth, death and funeral. A still photo can be made from a video tape thus giving parents a further opportunity to create photos. 'Still' photos and other mementoes can become part of the video too. A tape of the funeral is often valuable as parents may be still in shock and may not remember what was said and who came.

SAYING HELLO — CREATING A MEMENTO PACKAGE

Mementoes are all the parents will have left when their baby dies. There are no second chances to collect them. You have to organise a memento collection perfectly in order to avoid, possibly, a lifetime of regret.

Memories of the baby will come through the experience of pregnancy, birthing, the baby himself, the people providing care and the funeral. There are many opportunities for midwives to create opportunities for 'good' memories for the bereaved parents.

Encourage parents to remember with their senses — touching, smelling, and seeing their baby.

LATE PREGNANCY LOSS MEMORY CREATION LIST FOR PARENTS

(see also Chapter 1)

- Try to have a pair each of the baby's footprints and handprints. Remove ink with an alcohol wipe and damp cotton wool. Warn parents that not all of the ink will come off. Ink prints may be photocopied because the ink may smudge if you attempt to make multiple copies. Some hospitals use coloured shoe polish or washable pastel paint instead of ink.
- Place two name bands on the baby then take one off to give to the parents, leaving the other so that the baby doesn't get lost.
- Prepare baby name cards, written in calligraphy if possible, recording the baby's weight, length, head circumference, time of birth and time of death.
- Keep the disposable tape measure used to measure the baby.
- Use two cord clamps – keep one on the baby and offer the other to the parents.
- Put a lock of hair in a tiny cellophane bag held together with ribbon or stapled to a memento card. If you have a choice, take the hair from the back of the baby's head so it is not as noticeable. It may not be possible to cut a lock with scissors but might be possible to shave some 'fuzz' with a dry safety razor.
- Keep fingernail clippings.
- Make 'kiss' prints by placing lipstick on the baby's lips then pressing them to a card.
- Make a photocopy of the printout from any electronic fetal monitoring that has occurred during the pregnancy. Give the copy to the parents while retaining the original for the medical record.
- Many pathology departments carry out routine x-rays so copies can be offered to the parents.
- Make an outline sketch of the baby by drawing around the baby's body. Siblings can have outline drawings done at the same time and these can be kept in the same place. These give a concept of size.
- Press some of the flowers received.
- Parents, relatives and friends may offer a donation to a charitable organisation on behalf of the baby. Many organisations send thank you cards or recognise the donation in a year book. This record may be added to the memento package.

All the above can be made into a keepsake folder or album. Other mementoes may include:
- imprints of the baby's feet and/or hands in clay, plaster or 'mastic' (dentists use this), or a mould of the baby's face, feet or hands
- clothes the baby wore and/or the blanket the baby was wrapped in — in fact, anything that has touched the baby (see dummy/pacifier story below)
- soft leather shoes worn by the baby then dipped in gold or bronze to provide a three-dimensional memento.

We midwives are in a position to help parents create mementoes:
- Many nurseries keep diaries, often written as if the baby is talking, e.g. 'Today I had my first bath and a photo was taken.' If it is known that the baby will die it is probably even more important that such a diary is commenced, with pictures and milestones.
- Baby powder or scented bath water may create a scent memory. (In a slightly different but related vein, be aware that sense of smell seems to be heightened during stress, so you should avoid wearing strong perfume as this may detract from the parents creating a scent memory of their baby.)

One bereaved mother created a very special memento:

> *When we went to the funeral parlour to see our baby for the last time I was upset to see that Robert's lips had darkened and his mouth was slightly open. I explained to the funeral director that I had anticipated the opportunity to take more photos but that I didn't want photos of Robert looking that way. The funeral director suggested that I purchase a dummy/pacifier and take the photos with this in his mouth. After I had taken the photos I took the dummy home and subsequently had it dipped in gold. Now it is a very treasured memento which sits on the mantelpiece along with his photo.*

BAPTISM/BLESSING

The baptism or blessing of the baby provides another opportunity for memory creation. It is important that parents are offered the option of having their baby blessed or baptised and that this is arranged carefully and with sensitivity to their religious and cultural needs (see Appendix 5).

> *When the minister arrived to baptise our baby I really wish we had thought to bring in our family's baptismal cup from home. As it was he just used his cupped hand but it would have been much nicer if we had had the cup.*

It is a good idea for a baptismal cup or some other item used for baptism, e.g. a seashell, to be readily available. If a seashell is used it may be given to the parents as a memento along with a baptismal certificate and perhaps a candle.

RELATIVES AND FRIENDS

> *One of my main regrets is that none of my family and friends saw our baby. I really wish now that someone had suggested that we ask close family and friends in to see him, and hold him so they could know he was real and that he was beautiful.*

It may be helpful to discuss visiting arrangements with the bereaved parents. Some may choose no visitors at all whilst others may prefer open visiting. As a midwife caring for the family you are usually in a position to know if there have been any visitors. If there have not, it may be that they are staying away. It is certainly helpful to the grieving family if others in their circle of family and friends have seen and held the baby. Suggesting this to the bereaved family may prevent regrets later.

FORMS AND DOCUMENTS

Documents to do with the baby differ from state to state and country to country. However, some kind of notification of birth is usually required in late pregnancy. Parents may require assistance in completing the forms. A photocopy of the notification form may be given to the parents as a memento.

SUPPORT

Midwives are not usually trained counsellors. Therefore it is not appropriate for us to attempt to counsel. However, we have a crucial role in helping parents start on the road to recovery in the best possible way given the circumstances. Here are some of the things we can, and probably should, do.

- Offer parents options but avoid offering your own opinion.
- Think how to put things to parents. It is often difficult to know what to say to bereaved people. My advice is: when in doubt say nothing. Avoid clichés.
- Human touch may speak louder than words. Be aware of where you touch: to touch someone on the knee may be perceived as patronising; the area between the shoulder and elbow is generally considered a neutral area to touch as a way of conveying empathy to a person.
- Bereaved parents tend to follow your example so be aware of your body language as well as of what you say.
- Be honest; don't be afraid to show your emotions, but be careful how you express yourself.
- Keep to a minimum the number of staff who care for the family during their hospital stay and for the follow-up period. This means there will be extra pressure on the staff involved but it is best for the family.

LACTATION

I cried when it came in and I cried when it disappeared because it was a link with him.

Some mothers may not want any milk at all to remind them of their baby, others may wish to have the experience of their milk 'coming in' as a link to their baby.

Suppression with drugs, particularly bromocriptine, is used less these days but may still be used by some doctors after perinatal death. Midwives need to be aware of how this drug acts and warn mothers of the likely side effects.

Minimising breast engorgement without prescribed medication

- **Cabbage leaves:** Place the cold, washed, outer leaves of a cabbage in a binder or bra and replace them regularly, as soon as they become warm.

- **Cabbage gel** is a soothing, cooling, aloe vera-based gel containing peppermint oil, herbal infusions and cabbage extract. Its purpose is to cool and soothe the engorged breast. Used alone, it offers topical cooling to the skin. Used with cabbage leaves, as described above, it helps the leaves adhere more securely to the breast and often speeds up the relief of breast engorgement.

- **Sage drops:** An infusion of two teaspoons of sage in 50 ml of boiling water, steeped for 5–10 minutes may be taken up to three times a day, if tolerated (it may cause stomach upset). Sage should not be taken internally regularly for more than a week or two as it may harm the liver. It should be avoided by epileptics as it may trigger seizures.

- **Wheat germ extract** is thought to be a prolactin inhibitor. It is a fine, water-soluble powder that can be mixed or stirred into a variety of hot or cold drinks, or sprinkled over food.

- **Bind** the breasts firmly.

- **Ice:** Apply ice packs to axillary area of breasts for 20 minutes 4-6 times a day as needed.

Other lactation suppression support measures

- Administer analgesics as needed.
- Administer night sedation as needed.
- Encourage women to wear supportive, well-fitting bras continuously until lactation is suppressed.
- Advise women to avoid breast stimulation.
- Inform bereaved mothers of the signs and symptoms of mastitis (tell them and write the information down) and ask them to seek prompt medical attention should these occur.

CHECKLIST FOR DISCHARGE PLANNING

Going home is almost always difficult for the parents. Some bereaved parents may request early discharge, others may wish to stay for the usual length of stay. It is very important that parents do not feel pressured to leave early simply because their baby has died. Domiciliary midwifery services may be utilised for bereaved parents who elect for early discharge just as they would if the baby had lived. It is best if information for discharge is written down to back up what you tell the family.

Discharge planning should cover a number of topics.

- Inform the parents of where the baby will be, whether they will still be able to visit after they go home and whom they should contact if they wish to see their baby again. Some parents may wake in the middle of the night and desperately want to hold their baby. It should be possible to visit either the hospital or the funeral parlour even in the middle of the night, as both these places provide a 24-hour service. Prepare the parents for the fact that their baby will feel cold to touch and will probably have darkened lips.
- Provide information about whom to contact if they need to talk, including self-help support groups, social workers, chaplains etc.
- Give them support group information. Offer to make the first contact for them. Ask the couple if you can give the local support group their address for a newsletter and other printed literature to be sent.
- Offer a book list for suggested further reading.
- Make sure they understand what they might expect physically, e.g. lactation and lochia.
- Warn them about postpartum 'blues' and depression.
- Alert them to the possibility of hallucinations, vivid dreams, flashbacks and other sensory disturbances.
- Let them know what to expect from outside agencies, e.g. bills from the hospital, pathology laboratories, the obstetrician and others involved in the birth; unwelcome letters from promotional companies; calls from insurance salespeople etc.

- Make them aware of likely reactions from family and friends. Many bereaved parents find their family and friends less than supportive. This can drive a wedge into the friendship, which may be irreparable unless the parents realise that most of their family and friends cannot hope to understand the enormity of their loss and may therefore unintentionally hurt on a regular and long-term basis.
- Prepare them for likely triggers for grief, e.g. arriving home to the prepared nursery, hearing certain music, seeing a certain toy, other people's babies, pregnant tummies, living through anniversaries etc.
- Discuss contraception.
- Try to help them cope with entering the real world of pregnant tummies and happy babies.
- Notify the early childhood nurse to avoid distressing contact later.
- Parents whose baby has died in NICU may wish to visit the unit again. Provide information about who to contact to arrange this. Point out that the parents may need to prearrange the visit so that staff who cared for their baby are rostered on when the parents intend coming.

SAYING FAREWELL

They asked me if I wanted a hospital funeral and I didn't know what it meant so I agreed. It was a mass grave. I regret that no-one explained what a 'hospital funeral' meant.

The newly bereaved parents are likely to be young, with limited experience of death. For many, their dead child may be the first dead person they have ever seen. Most will not have had the sole responsibility of organising a funeral before. Some may not have any idea where to start. A funeral director will be able to assist them, but you may help them by starting them thinking about what kind of ceremony they would like to have to say goodbye appropriately to their baby.

The funeral is another time for memory creation. If you are asked, suggest that the funeral happens later rather than sooner. A delay will allow parents time to plan a more meaningful funeral for their baby. The decisions the parents make in connection with the funeral will be the last parenting decisions they make for this child. Midwives are often asked what kinds of things other parents have found meaningful in this situation.

CREATING A MEMORABLE FUNERAL

- Someone from the family may wish to carry the tiny casket — father and/or siblings, or perhaps grandparents.
- The baby can be cuddled throughout the funeral and then placed in the coffin. Some parents have not had the opportunity to hold their baby. A closed coffin funeral can lead the parents to wonder later if their baby was really inside the coffin.
- Flower arrangements can be in the shape of a teddy bear, an angel or some other childhood image.
- Balloons in appropriate colours or shapes can be tied to the casket whilst the funeral is taking place, then let go prior to the committal or kept, at the parents' wish.
- People who come can place an article of childhood or other memento with the baby. These can be buried with the baby or placed with the ashes.
- Parents can buy a piece of jewellery in memory of their baby. Some mothers may buy a pair of earrings then place one in the coffin and keep the other.
- A photo of the family can be buried/cremated with the baby.
- The baby can wear a name bracelet, in fact the whole family may choose to wear bracelets engraved with the baby's name.
- The casket does not have to be white, neither does the lining fabric. Parents can choose whatever colour or lining fabric they wish.
- Children from the family can 'decorate' the outside of the coffin by drawing pictures or making handprints for their dead sibling.
- Stories, poems or prayers written to the baby or for the baby can be read and then placed in the coffin.
- If the baby is cremated a special container can be purchased for the ashes — an appropriate wood, pottery, or stone box, or a metal (perhaps silver) vessel which can be engraved as an 'urn' for the baby. Let parents know what size vessel to purchase so that the baby's ashes actually fit.
- Some parents choose a 'theme' for their baby's funeral — angels, teddy bears, rosebuds etc. — then everything to do with the funeral can be connected by the theme. For example, if the rosebud theme were

chosen the parents may wear a rosebud which could be later pressed or dried; the flowers placed on the casket could be rosebuds; the order of service may have a rosebud printed on it; balloons may have rosebuds embossed on them.

- A basket of flowers can be provided so that every person at the funeral can either place a flower on the casket or take a flower home.
- Most undertakers provide an attendance list of signatures of people at the funeral. This, together with a copy of the order of service, can be kept with other mementoes.
- The handles and name plate are usually removed from a coffin prior to cremation. They can be kept as a keepsake with other mementoes.
- Music for the service may include nursery rhymes, lullabies etc.
- Include surviving children from the family in the funeral service and invite children of family and friends to be there too. However, it is a good idea to organise another adult to care for the children if they become unsettled so that parents are not rushed through their farewell to their baby.
- A memorial service can be held in addition to or instead of a funeral.

If you were involved in the couple's care when their baby was stillborn, or provided care for their sick/dying neonate, you may consider going to the baby's funeral. It is wise to ask first, but many parents will appreciate your attendance.

FOLLOW-UP

We also got a sympathy card from the hospital, personally signed by the doctors and nurses who had cared for me.

Once home many parents find that the support they need is not available for as long as they need (Barkway, 1996).

Planned follow-up after the death of a baby can improve general health outcomes for parents, particularly those considered to be at risk (Murray and Murray, 1994). Hospitals generally don't have the funding for ongoing support however it is important that some follow-up is included in the care of bereaved parents (especially if they go home early) including general support and assessment, referral, and early detection of problems. A midwife involved in the delivery and after care has a special link to these parents and should be involved in follow-up.

It is ideal for contact to continue at regular intervals for the first year following the bereavement. Allow the parents to control the level of their follow-up. Leave a telephone contact and ask for their telephone number in return. The midwife who is to be involved in the follow-up should have a meeting with the parents prior to discharge to gain permission to visit them at home and arrange times when phone contact can be made.

The ideal contact pattern is:
- several times in the first few weeks for emotional support and physical assessment
- six weeks after the birth for a postnatal check (usually done by a doctor); a check on the couple's emotional and physical health; discussion of the autopsy, recurrence risks and/or referral for genetic counselling; likely care in future pregnancies; and referral to a support group
- at 3–6 months for a general chat and the opportunity for parents to ask questions
- on the 12-month anniversary — face-to-face or telephone contact and/or send a card.

In addition
- Send a letter to the GP including information gained from the six-week check, together with relevant further investigations, referrals and suggestions for management of future pregnancies.
- If the loss was a neonatal death a follow-up appointment with the neonatologist is also usual.

What do you do during contact?

If you are visiting the parents in their home, tell them why you are there and how long you will stay (less than an hour) as they may be unsure as to the purpose of your visit. Allow them to talk about what has happened and ask questions if they wish. It is helpful if you just listen. Provide a time to answer questions.

Specifically ask about sleep. Many bereaved parents find it very hard to sleep. Reassure them that this is normal. They may require sedatives but it is not the best option. Sleeping tablets do not usually provide a natural sleep and most people do not wake feeling refreshed. Many bereaved parents find that sleeping tablets do not work. If parents can be reassured that insomnia is a very normal part of grief, that it will settle and they will eventually be able to sleep peacefully again, then their requirements for artificial assistance may be limited.

REFERENCES

Barkway P (1996): Parents' experience after Perinatal death. Paper presented to SANDS 6th National Conference, Adelaide, October 1996.

Lloyd Karon (1992): *A Part of You Dies.* Video produced and directed by Karon Lloyd and available from her at PO Box 263, Blaxland, NSW 2774.

McPhee A (1995): Untitled paper presented to SANDS seminar, 'Perinatal Death: Implications for the Caring Professions.' Adelaide.

Moscarello R (1989): Perinatal Bereavement Support Service: Three-year review. *Journal of Palliative Care* 5 (4): 12–18.

Murray J, Murray M (1994): *When the Dream Is Shattered.* Adelaide: Lutheran Publishing House.

Thearle MJ, Gregory HJ (1992): Evolution of bereavement counselling in sudden infant death syndrome, neonatal death and stillbirth. *Paediatr Child Health* 28 (3) June: 204–209.

Wright B (1993): *Caring in Crisis.* Edinburgh: Churchill Livingstone.

INTERESTING RESEARCH ARTICLES

Bluglass K (1992):The sudden infant death — psychological consequences and role of the medical team. *Annales Nestlé* 50: 81.

Bourne S, Lewis E (1991): Perinatal bereavement: A milestone and some new dangers *BMJ* 302, 18 May: 1167–8.

Calhoun LK (1994): Parents' perceptions of nursing support following neonatal loss. *Journal of Perinatal and Neonatal Nursing* 8 (2): 57–62.

Dyregrov A (1990): Parental reactions to the loss of an infant child: A review. *Scand Journal of Psych* 31: 266-280.

Kavanaugh K (1997): Parents' experience surrounding the death of a new-born whose birth is at the margin of viability. *JOGNN* Jan./Feb.: 43–51.

Leon I (1992): Perinatal loss: A critique of current hospital practices. *Clinical Paediatrics* 31: 366-374.

Mander R (1991): Midwifery care of the grieving mother — how the decisions are made. *Midwifery* 7 (3): 133-42.

Primeau M, Lamb J (1995): When a baby dies: Rights of the baby and parents. *JOGNN* 24 (3): 206-8.

Schwab R (1996): Gender differences in parental grief. *Death Studies* 20: 103-113.

Sweeney M (1997):The value of a family centered approach in the NICU and PICU: One family's perspective. *Pediatric Nursing* 23: 1.

RECOMMENDED READING

Arnold J, Gemma P (1994): *A Child Dies, A Portrait of Family Grief* 2nd edn. Philadelphia: The Charles Press.

Crowther R, Brabin P (1986): *Your Baby Has Died.* Melbourne: SANDS Victoria.

De Frain J (1991): *Stillborn: The Invisible Death.* Lexington: Heath/Lexington Books.

Fumia M (1990): *A Child at Dawn, the Healing of a Memory.* Notre Dame: Arreman's Press.

Kohn I, Moffitt P-L (1993): *A Silent Sorrow, Pregnancy Loss. Guidance and Support for You and Your Family.* New York: Bantam Press.

Lord JD (1987): *When a Baby Suddenly Dies.* Melbourne: Hill of Content.

Schwiebert P, Kirk P (1985): *When Hello Means Goodbye.* Portland: Perinatal Loss.

Stewart A, Dent A (1994): *At a Loss.* London: Bailliere Tindall.

Vredevelt P (1995): *Empty Arms.* Sisters: Multnomah Press.

CHAPTER 4

LOSS IN A MULTIPLE PREGNANCY

I didn't see 'one baby', I saw 'not two'.
(Kollantai, 1994)

With apologies to parents of higher multiples, in this chapter I have referred to multiples generally as 'twins', purely for ease of writing and reading.

DEFINITION

A study by Chitrit et al. (1999) found the perinatal mortality rate in twin pregnancy is 7-8 times higher than in singleton pregnancy. They also found that extreme prematurity accounted for nearly half of the perinatal death rate in twins.

Expectant parents of twins often feel special. Frequently family and friends show extraordinary interest in the couple and 'fuss' over the growing pregnancy. When one or more babies dies, either during the pregnancy or in the perinatal period, the parents lose not only their baby/ies but their 'specialness'. They lose both a baby and a twin.

Midwives caring for families who have lost a twin must include in their care all the same routines as when a singleton baby dies, and must carry out 'multiple-specific' practices as well.

BREAKING BAD NEWS

> The phrase 'Well at least you've still got a baby' rang in my ears for weeks, even months! (Schulz, 1998)

It is important to break bad news in a tactful, sympathetic manner. Avoid implying that the couple are in any way lucky to have a surviving baby. The bereaved parents do not usually feel fortunate that one of their twins has lived. Most commonly they feel distressed that one of their babies has died.

SUPPORT WHILE IN HOSPITAL AFTER BAD NEWS IS BROKEN

> The nursing staff had no idea what to do with me. They originally put me in a room with another woman who was carrying twins — except hers were both alive! I felt so angry, hurt and cheated! I was amazed that the staff could be so insensitive to my situation. (Schulz, 1998)

If the mother needs to be hospitalised for any reason then it is best to ask the mother where in the antenatal ward she would like to be situated. Some may wish to be with other mothers who have living twins, others may wish to avoid these mothers altogether.

LIVING WITH THE LOSS

> It was difficult to cope with the fact that my body was slowly destroying one of the most precious gifts that I had ever received and I could do absolutely nothing about it . . . I had to force myself to eat. If I didn't eat the other baby might die too. It is very difficult. With each mouthful large tears slid silently down my cheeks. I felt so alone. (Schulz, 1998)

Mothers who have to continue a pregnancy with both a living baby and a dead baby are embroiled in a situation over which they have no control.

Grief can be overwhelming and pressing, the need to focus on the living baby can be just as overwhelming. Coping with both at the same time is a quite dreadful situation in which to try to live. It is paramount that staff caring for the mother for the remainder of her pregnancy exhibit understanding and compassion. This situation can be eased by acknowledging what has happened and continuing to allow the parents the opportunity to talk about both of their babies.

> I have an ultrasound downstairs. I ask the staff about my dead baby but no-one knows what to say . . . The scan is good — if you could call it that. The live baby is growing well and strong. The other baby is just a still grey mass on the screen . . . I love that still grey mass! (Schulz, 1998)

THE BIRTH

> I don't look forward to the delivery because although I will have my live baby, the doctors will take the other one away. It is comforting still having the baby attached inside of me. At least I can still hold onto the both of them — for just a bit longer. (Schulz, 1998)

As delivery of the living baby approaches, the mother may feel reluctant to birth. If the birth is to be vaginal midwives need to take into account the situation, especially if there is any unexpected delay in the progress of labour. If such a delay occurs then take the time to talk to the mother about what will happen after the birth. Especially encourage opportunities to see and hold both babies together.

> *I would have liked to have had a mirror so I could see the birth. The midwife just assumed that I wouldn't want to.*

It is wise not to assume that the 'normal' trappings associated with a vaginal delivery are not wanted because one of the babies is expected to be stillborn.

> After the babies are born each baby should be seen and held for as long as desired and more than once if desired, regardless of the condition of the baby or the mother, or of any survivors. (CLIMB, 1993)

It is ideal to hold the babies together. If this is not possible then at least see them side by side or take a photo of them hugging or touching hands.

MEETING THE BABIES

> One unthinking student midwife informed me that my baby might resemble a 'piece of meat' . . . As I lay in the recovery ward, I noticed my husband standing near a wall, speaking to a nurse holding a small bundle. I knew it was Megan! Rhys had been placed in a humid-crib to ensure that his body temperature was stabilised, so I knew that they had my daughter. I felt so torn, and so very, very frightened! I desperately wanted to see my only daughter, to hold her and show how much love I had for her, but the words of the student midwife kept floating in my exhausted mind. I did not want to look at a piece of meat wrapped in a baby blanket! . . .
>
> As I looked up, my eyes met those of my husband. He was calm and serene . . . 'Trust me,' he said 'it's okay.' I knew then that it was all right to look at the bundle that he now held in his arms. And I was so glad I did! Megan was mine, and she was beautiful! She looked like a baby, except that she had to be wrapped extremely carefully because her body was so soft and spongy.
>
> This was my only chance to hold her, and to say 'hello' and 'goodbye'.
> (Schulz, 1996)

It is difficult to predict parents' reaction to seeing a baby who has been dead in utero for some time. Megan had been dead for five weeks and yet Lynne says:

> I felt so proud of her — my heart went out to her. 'I love you, Megan — goodbye my darling.' They were the only words that I could think of as I looked into her empty, puppy-like eyes. I was not repulsed, I was not disgusted, I was proud!
> (Schulz, 1998)

However Angela said:

> *I did not want to see my baby. He had been dead for a couple of months and I really didn't want to see him but the midwife just kept insisting until I relented. It was a terrible thing. My baby looked a horrible colour. Still to this day (six years later) I cannot look at anything that colour without getting a vivid flashback. His pathetic little form still haunts my nightmares . . . it took me a LONG time to forgive that midwife. Now I can say I am grateful for the opportunity to see and cuddle my baby but it took me three years to get to the point where I could even say that. Up until then I would have cheerfully murdered her if I had seen her in the street.*

Ari's mother was not 'allowed' to see her baby. Although she accepted her midwife's decision, she would still have appreciated a careful description of her baby:

> *I was not allowed to see my daughter. The midwife told me that my daughter was decomposed (she'd been gone for 12 weeks prior to birth), and that her appearance would likely be upsetting to us. But I would have liked the midwife to have told us 'She has lots of dark hair' or 'She has blue eyes like her brother' or even 'She has your nose'. It might have given me at least part of a face to put with the 'what-ifs' and 'what-might-have-beens'.*

(In this situation it may have been possible to take a close-up photo, perhaps even with black and white film, of a part of the baby, e.g. a foot or a hand, in order to give the parents at least something to show that they are parents of twins.)

How can midwives help parents to meet both babies if one has been dead in utero for some time? I believe the answer is not to force, but to let the parent guide you. Lynne just needed reassurance that it was OK to look by someone who had already seen her baby. She was pleased and relieved she did. Angela may have benefited from a full and frank description of her baby's appearance including the baby's colour. Ari's mum may have benefited from being given a choice rather than the assumption being made for her that she didn't want to look just because the midwife didn't think it was appropriate. She too may have benefited from a full description of her baby.

THE LIVING AND THE DEAD

> When one twin dies perinatally, mothers and fathers have a very confusing, ambivalent induction into new parenthood. Congratulations and condolences, birth and death announcements, baptismal gowns and caskets are all a part of the first few postpartum weeks. While trying to attach to the surviving twin, parents are also experiencing the need to grieve the dead twin. (Swanson Kauffman, 1988)

Parents may be torn between grieving for the twin who died and looking after the surviving twin. It is very difficult for such parents to manage to do both adequately. They may either appear to be 'coping well' and look after their surviving twin or they may 'go to pieces' and concentrate on mourning at the expense of the surviving twin. A few parents may be able to cope with both, as this mother describes:

> I had to acknowledge the reality of the situation. I had two babies. I was one
> person, and, as with two living twins, I could only give time to one baby at a
> time. I decided Laura would forgive me when I was openly happy with David.
> David would understand when I needed grieving time for Laura. He probably
> needed some grieving time for Laura too! It was this understanding and
> forgiveness that allowed me to give each of them the time they needed.
> (Wegner-Hay, 1988)

If a choice is to be made as to which of their babies parents spend time with,
encourage them to spend time with their dead or dying infant. The surviving
twin will have a lifetime of attention and parenting whereas the parents have
only a very brief opportunity to parent their dead or dying baby. Help, and allow
the parents to spend time with their dead or dying baby without being made
to feel guilty in any way. Explain why you are encouraging such an uneven
division of their time.

> They acted as if my surviving twin was my main baby, and Andrew was at
> most a nice extra that didn't quite work out. (WiSSPERS, 1994)

It is most important for midwives to acknowledge these parents as parents of
twins. It is not helpful to imply in any way that the parents 'wouldn't have
wanted twins in any case' or that 'one baby is sufficient to parent'.

> Later that evening I have a strong desire to see my babies, but I dare not ask
> anyone. I have tubes everywhere, every part of me aches and I feel so sick.
> Later, Rhys is brought upstairs from recovery to share my room and my life —
> no-one talks about Megan. (Schulz 1998)

Bereaved parents of twins often have limited opportunities to see, photograph
and cuddle their babies together. Parents who have had little or no contact with
their babies together will usually regret this lost opportunity. Midwives can
assist the parents to avoid such later regrets by offering, on more than one
occasion, another cuddle with both babies.

If one or more babies dies from a set of triplets or higher then it may be
tempting to see this as a blessing for the parents. After all, one may ask, who can
cope with three babies at once anyway? However, it is important —
irrespective of how many died, how many lived, or when the death occurred
(even if early in the pregnancy) — to allow the parents to acknowledge and
grieve for their baby/ies who died. It is really important to acknowledge the
parents as parents of twins and to talk about the dead baby just as you would
if it were a singleton death.

CREATING MEMORIES

> Experiencing our babies together after birth, in whatever way possible, has an immeasurable positive impact on long-term healing, marriage, and parenting of other children. (WiSSPERS, 1994)

Everything I have already written about memory creation applies to twins. However, special consideration needs to be given to creating mementoes of twins, one of whom is living, the other dead.

> The only pictures we have of our daughter are a poor quality instant snapshot, just after the birth, and a very clear picture of her after the autopsy. (Schulz, 1996)

Photos taken of the twins separately and together will assist parents to see their babies as individuals.

> *The social worker sent two clear photos taken before the autopsy, but it wasn't the same thing as if we had been encouraged to take our own.*

Encourage the parents to take some photos themselves as this may assist them in later memory recall.

> *I would have liked some photos of us holding our baby and pictures of our twins together. I feel very sad. It's hard to not have anything that shows people that I am the mother of twins.*

Hold the babies at the same time, ideally one in each arm, to have a photo of them together. Take at least one photo of the twins together, touching hands. If circumstances do not allow the twins to be photographed together then parents may still have their babies sketched together in one print.

Other items outlined in the previous chapter should be collected from both babies to enable the parents to show they are parents of twins.

BREASTFEEDING THE SURVIVING TWIN

> Every time that I breastfed Rhys, all I could think of was 'poor little Megan' . . . poor Rhys, the last thing he needed was a crying woman every time he wanted a feed!
>
> Other complications, such as cracked bleeding nipples, only added further strain to the whole situation. I endured this for five days, and after a lot of tears, and long-distance phone calls to Luke at home, and quizzing the nursing staff, who weren't allowed to support bottle feeding, I made the decision to bottle feed. I was now depressed about Megan, as well as feeling like the 'World's Biggest Failure' for no longer breastfeeding. (Schulz, 1998)

It is well known that high levels of anxiety usually impact on the ability to breastfeed successfully. The 'let-down' or 'draught' reflex is inhibited by stress, as is the release of the hormone relaxin. Careful management of the initiation of breastfeeding, coupled with counselling from a trained counsellor, may assist bereaved mothers of twins to initiate and maintain breastfeeding successfully.

A SPECIAL SITUATION

> Some families may encounter a most difficult circumstance when there is a twin or multiple gestation pregnancy and one of the unborn babies is found to have an abnormality. (SAFDA, 1995)

In this situation, the parents may be offered selective termination. Parents who take up this option in early pregnancy may still face grief and doubt at the live birth of their surviving baby. Laura's mother describes how she alleviated her 'remorse and nagging doubts':

> A friend suggested I obtain my medical records and call Dr Nelson, who had been there when Laura died. I found it amazingly easy to retrieve my records. Reading the reports was painful but strangely reassuring. Laura had been very sick. Her condition was laid out for me in black and white. I read those records many times, so I could know what ailed my daughter and why death was inevitable for her. (Wegner-Hay, 1998)

DISCHARGE PREPARATION

> The first few weeks at home felt strange. When I first walked into my house after being away for almost two months, it was as though I had forgotten something. I was carrying one baby, yet it seemed only natural that I should be holding another. Whenever I changed one nappy, I sometimes turned to pick up another nappy for the next baby, except there was no baby there! It seemed odd to be doing things for just one, when my mind had trained itself somehow to automatically account for two! I did begin to wonder whether I was slowly losing my sanity! (Schulz, 1998)

Lynne's experiences are not unique. Midwives would do well to warn bereaved parents of the likelihood of such experiences occurring so bereaved parents are less likely to question their sanity.

LONGER-TERM ISSUES

> We love Rhys, but our hearts ache for Megan. (Schulz, 1998)

Coping with the demands of the surviving baby gives the parents precious little time to grieve. When a baby dies there are always 'reminder' days which may be difficult and painful.

> With the loss of a twin, however, the actual number of 'occasions' are increased exponentially by witnessing growth markers in the surviving twin . . . the surviving twin is, ironically, the never-ending reminder of what could have been. (Swanson-Kauffman, 1988)

One way of coping with the 'reminder days' is to make time for both babies in the day.

Bereaved parents of twins may benefit from:
- having one ceremony incorporating both a baptism and a memorial service
- permitting themselves to feel sad on days when the surviving twin reaches significant milestones
- celebrating one twin's birthday and, at the same time, commemorating the lives of both babies; for example, letting go the balloons used at the birthday party can mark the anniversary, thus allowing the parents the freedom to acknowledge both babies rather than feeling as if they are leaving one baby out

- following a suggestion from this parent:

  > *We decided that we would mourn Giana's passing the day that we found out that she had passed away, August 11th, so as not to ruin Kira's birthday. And we have stuck to that.*

A perfect baby is a dead baby. The living baby may be fretful or difficult to manage and the parents may find themselves wondering if the other baby would have been as 'difficult'. They may need to be reassured that it is okay to think that their dead baby may have been a better baby.

Bereaved parents of twins may be extraordinarily fearful of losing their surviving twin. They have lost their naiveté. They now know that pregnancies are lost, babies do die. It happened to them and they may fear it could happen again. Health professionals caring for such parents need to understand and accept their fear. Avoid telling them that 'everything will be all right' Instead, offer them practical ways of overcoming their fear. Home monitoring may be an option. One mother of a surviving triplet monitored the baby at home for several months because she was so afraid she would lose all her babies. You may also suggest the baby sleeps in the same room as the parents. Of course some babies do die even if they are monitored and/or in the same room as their parents. However, if such a calamity were to occur, the parents may feel they had endeavoured to avoid it by doing all within their power. A mother of two surviving triplets expresses her feelings this way:

  > *I have a hard time dealing with joys of motherhood because it seems the more I am happy about their growths and achievements the more saddened I am because there should be a third one saying her ABC and giggling at the Walt Disney film that they are seeing for the third time that week. I feel such a void. I know that they have a guardian angel by them at all times, but sometimes I wish I could see that angel's smile.*

Parents of a surviving same-sex twin may wish to know if their twins were identical. This can be important to how the parents 'picture' the babies.

> Most of us do not expect to ever be pregnant with twins again. No-one can say 'Well, next year I'll have my subsequent twins.' (WiSSPERS, 1994)

It is important to acknowledge that bereaved parents of twins may wish to plan not only another pregnancy but also another multiple pregnancy. Whilst most will realise how unlikely another multiple pregnancy is, some may need careful counselling to resolve their grief over the loss of twinship for their child and themselves:

> No matter how many more children I may have my son will still not have his twin brother. (WiSSPERS, 1994)

SUPPORT

> Multiple birth support group visited me at 28 weeks. I told the lady that one baby might die and she disappeared out the door! (Schulz, 1998)

Bereaved parents may find it difficult to gain the ongoing support and understanding they need. They may feel equally out of place in a twins' support meeting as in a support meeting for those who have experienced the loss of a singleton baby. Some areas have a support group specifically to cater for loss in multiple pregnancy. This situation is ideal but unfortunately not very common. Counselling from a trained counsellor may be the best situation for those without peer support.

> I talked to the social worker and the funeral parlour director. They were the only people interested in my dead child. The midwives only acknowledged the living child. (Schulz, 1998)

SAYING GOODBYE

Parents may have to consider delaying the funeral for their baby if the outcome for the remaining baby is uncertain. Some parents prefer not to wait, preferring to be optimistic. Others will want to wait, especially if the situation is critical and they choose to have their babies buried together. If the parents choose to delay the funeral because their surviving baby is gravely ill then they will, of course, need extra support and understanding during this time.

> *I watched them die one after another. I started to wonder if I would get to take any home.*   (mother of sextuplets)

If the surviving baby is well and expected to live, the parents may wish to plan a joint baptism/funeral.

> We decided to have our daughter Sophie baptised at her brother Teddy's memorial service, as a way of celebrating their twinship and as the last event they could be part of 'together'. (Fleischer, 1988)

THINGS YOU SHOULD NEVER SAY TO A PARENT WHO HAS LOST A TWIN

- 'At least you have the other twin.'

  No-one replaces anyone, not even a genetically identical person born at exactly the same time. (WiSSPERS, 1994)

  While the bereaved parent is usually grateful for the surviving twin, nothing can take away the pain of losing a baby. The baby who died was not an 'extra' or a 'spare' baby, the baby lived (if only in utero) and breathed (if born alive.) When someone loses a parent, no-one would dare say to them 'Well, at least you still have your other parent.' Just like parents, babies are not interchangeable!

- 'You can always have another baby.'
  This cannot be assumed. If the parents have undergone fertility treatment, pregnancy may not ever happen again. Even if it does, the chances of having twins again are very remote. Parents whose twin dies lose not only the baby but the special twinship that exists between twins. The surviving child may grow up as an only child and this may be especially painful when the parents know their child did not start out life alone, that they should have a twin as they grow up.

- 'It was God's will.'
  God does not purposely take babies away from their families. Nor is this a punishment for something the bereaved parents did. What could they do that was so bad that God would punish them by taking the life of their child? Nothing! God doesn't work that way! This falls into the category of 'stuff happens'.

- 'If you had to lose him, at least it happened now instead of after you had really gotten attached to him'.
  Parents, particularly mothers, become attached to their babies very early in pregnancy. Grief after loss in pregnancy can be intense because you don't get the opportunity to make many memories. Memories and reminiscing help in the grief process. If memories are few, then the grief is more painful not less. One mother said:

> *We had 24 short days with Zachary. I would have treasured even one more hour with him.*

- 'The one you have keeps you up all night and demands all of your attention, how would you have managed having two?'
  People who say this fail to understand just how difficult it is to look after one baby while you are grieving for the other. Most bereaved parents of twins probably feel that they would have managed better with a few extra sleepless nights and frazzled days than the constant grief and painful reminders. Moreover, as the years go by, anniversaries hurt and remind. The first smile; the first day of crawling, walking, riding a bike, being at school all happen to the surviving twin, and as each milestone passes, the bereaved parents wonder what it would have been like with two

REFERENCES

Chitrit Y, Filidori M, Pons JC, Duyme M, Papiernik E (1999): Perinatal mortality in twin pregnancies: a 3-year analysis in Seine Saint-Denis (France). *Eur J Obstet Gynecol Reprod Biol* Sept. 86 (1): 23–8.

CLIMB (Centre for Loss in Multiple Birth) Pamphlet (1993): *Multiple Loss and the Hospital Caregiver*. Palmer: CLIMB.

Fleischer L (1988): When One Twin Dies. In: Lamb JM (ed.): *Bittersweet: Hello/Goodbye. A resource in planning farewell rituals when a baby dies*. St Charles: National SHARE Office.

Kollantai J (1994): The emotional impact of stillbirth in a multiple pregnancy. *WiSSPERS* (Wisconsin Stillbirth Support Newsletter)1 (3) Spring.

SAFDA (Support After Fetal Diagnosis of Abnormality) (1995): *Diagnosis of Abnormality in an Unborn Baby. The Impact, Options and Afterwards*. Sydney: NSW Genetics Education Program.

Schulz L (1998): *The Diary*. Adelaide: Cleverclogs Independent Publishers.

Schulz L (1996): Sharing Experience of Losing a Twin. Paper presented to SANDS 6th National Conference, Adelaide, October 1996.

Swanson-Kauffman K (1988): There should have been two: Nursing care of parents experiencing the perinatal death of a twin. *J Perinat Neonatal Nursing* 2 (2): 78–86.

Wegner-Hay M (1998): *Embracing Laura.* Omaha: Centering Corporation.

INTERESTING RESEARCH ARTICLES

Lewis E, Bryan E (1988): Management of perinatal loss of a twin. *BMJ* 297: 1321.

Janssen HJ et al. (1996): Controlled prospective study on the mental health of women following pregnancy loss. *Am J Psychiatry* 153 (2) Feb.: 226–230.

RECOMMENDED READING

Case Betty Jean (1993): *Living without Your Twin.* Portland: Tibbutt Pub.

Centering Vignette (1984): *Death of an Infant Twin.* Omaha: Centering Corporation.

Galinsky H (1976): *Beginnings.* Boston: Houghton Mifflin.

Noble E (1991): *Having Twins: A Parent's Guide to Pregnancy, Birth and Early Childhood* 2nd edn. Boston: Houghton Mifflin Co.

Woodward J (1998): *The Lone Twin: Understanding Twin Bereavement and Loss.* London: Free Assn Books.

CHAPTER 5

SUBSEQUENT PREGNANCY

There was a time when pregnancy equalled baby to me, but now pregnancy equals grief, death, emotional and physical pain, and failure.

(Personal communication)

A TENTATIVE PREGNANCY

In her book *The Tentative Pregnancy* Barbara Katz Rothman (1988) describes a 'tentative' pregnancy as one where the pregnant woman says to herself 'If everything is okay I will have a baby.' Pregnancy after the loss of a baby is often 'tentative'.

Many bereaved parents find, whilst wanting to be pregnant, they do not feel 'happy' during the pregnancy. Anxiety and fear coupled with distrust of the medical community and disbelief that their bodies can keep a baby safe are common. Many bereaved mothers will be anxious. They may not trust you when you try to reassure them that aches and pains they are experiencing are 'normal' in pregnancy. In fact, the next pregnancy is often an emotional minefield because, no matter how long it has been since the previous loss, most families begin the pregnancy still grieving for the baby who died. Midwives caring for families enduring a subsequent pregnancy after the death of a baby need to realise the tentative nature of the pregnancy for the family and adapt their management accordingly.

OBSTETRIC OUTCOME

> For me as an individual woman facing another pregnancy, the risk at the
> emotional level is simply 50%. That is, a bad outcome either will happen again
> or it won't. (SAFDA, 1995)

There is much research which suggests that subsequent pregnancy after the
death of a baby is likely to result in a 'worse' obstetric and neonatal outcome.
Crowther (1995) retrospectively studied a group of women with a history of a
previous stillbirth or neonatal death, comparing their obstetric outcome with a
control group who were matched for age, parity, and socioeconomic status. The
index group were statistically more likely to:
- be admitted to hospital during their pregnancy (46% vs 26%)
- have medical complications (58% vs 34%)
- be delivered prematurely (16%vs 8%)
- be delivered by Caesarean section (22% vs 9%).

Their babies were more likely to:
- have complications (28.8% vs 20.4%)
- be of low birthweight (14% vs 7%)
- require intubation (11% vs 5%)
- be admitted to the special care baby unit(13%vs 7%).

The study also noted a high degree of medical intervention in the absence of
clear medical indication.

Hence, a woman enduring a subsequent pregnancy after the death of a baby
warrants special attention from the midwives caring for her.

THE MIDWIFE'S ROLE IN SUBSEQUENT PREGNANCY

There are a number of ways that you can provide for families to enable them to
better cope with the stresses and strains of a subsequent pregnancy. It is good
to be positive with women, especially when they feel negative, but don't go
overboard by trying to guarantee them a live, healthy baby. Give them hope
without false reassurance.

Antenatal care

I was more assertive with all those involved in my antenatal, delivery and postnatal care. After the trauma I had been through I felt I had every right to demand particular things that I felt were important to me and my baby. (Warland and Warland, 1996)

It is common for bereaved parents to want their care to be different in their subsequent pregnancy; this may include changing doctors and hospitals. The parents may need concrete evidence that this pregnancy is different. They may want to know how it will be managed differently and what they can do differently.

Many families who have endured the loss of a baby will be more assertive and perhaps even demanding. This is both natural and understandable. The kind of support services midwives can offer are:

- opportunities to discuss issues or answer questions about the previous pregnancy
- clear explanations of the care and support the parents will receive, best presented in written form
- an outline of tests and procedures likely to be offered in this pregnancy, what they are for and why they are suggested
- access to continuity of a health care provider who is both willing and able to reassure parents
- a childbirth education program specifically for bereaved parents undergoing a subsequent pregnancy
- contact with a self-help group or other families who are enduring a subsequent pregnancy.

Anniversaries

It is common for bereaved couples to present with problems on anniversary dates. Reading the case notes may provide a clue to the current presenting problem. If this pregnancy is at or around the gestational age of their previous loss, if it is the same month or day of their previous loss or the presenting symptoms are the same or similar to what happened last time, then the presenting problem may be connected to anxiety from the previous loss. The anniversary may not be immediately obvious, e.g. the last baby may have died at Easter and Easter may be approaching, or the last baby may have died a week after some kind of natural disaster and the same kind of disaster has just recurred. It may not be possible to pinpoint every possible anniversary but with careful history taking and documentation many of the most likely anniversary times should be noted in the case record.

The woman may present to you with:
- decreased fetal movement
- fear of the baby being dead
- fear of ruptured membranes
- contractions
- anxiety attacks
- vague feelings that she cannot articulate.

Care needs to be taken to take the couple seriously when they present and to do everything within your power to set their minds at rest.

Communication

Be very careful when you are communicating with bereaved parents during a subsequent pregnancy. Communication breakdown can be common between health professional and lay person at the best of times, and with anxiety and grief clouding the issue, some understanding may be lost. Provide families with written information and encourage the woman to attend all her visits with a support person who will be better able to listen carefully and remind the woman later about what was said.

Tests, screens, procedures and routines

> If this pregnancy was to end tragically too there is little my doctor or anyone could do to prevent it. (Warland and Warland, 1996)

We have many prenatal tests, procedures and routines at our disposal yet, largely, medical science still cannot predict pregnancy loss or do very much to save a baby in trouble prior to the age of viability. Bereaved parents know this. Some may ask for every test known to mankind in order to reassure themselves that everything that can be done for their baby is being done. Others may feel there is little point in performing tests and screens if the outcome of the pregnancy will be unaffected by the results. Parents with a history of fetal abnormality may be especially fearful or anxious. Health professionals need to be aware of these likely feelings. Ask the family how they feel about prenatal tests and, where possible, accommodate the family's requests. Many parents in a subsequent pregnancy will be anxious. Reassurance may be simply provided by offering fetal kick charts in order to allow the mother to tune into her baby. CTG (electronic fetal monitoring) may also provide temporary relief from stress.

ANTENATAL VISIT CHECKLIST

First visit, approximately 8–12 weeks

- Discuss the family's support network. Make suggestions if the parents do not feel well supported.
- Ask about anxiety, ambivalence and/or excitement level.
- Ask if the parents wish you to mention/not mention their dead baby, including anniversary times.
- Discuss the need for 'debriefing', i.e. visiting the labour ward or the nursery prior to the new baby's birth.
- If the baby who died was born at the same hospital, there may be rooms, corridors or lifts which hold difficult memories for the couple and may be best avoided. Ask if this is so and make an entry in the case notes.

Subsequent visits

- Discuss ongoing need for support and ways of coping with anxiety.
- *8 weeks and on:* Offer the opportunity to listen to the fetal heart.
- *16 weeks — blood tests:* Give information on all prenatal testing including risks, false positives and likely outcomes.
- *18–20 weeks:* If diagnostic ultrasound is offered routinely, suggest a support person accompany the woman to the ultrasound. (Ultrasonography may be particularly stressful if it was used to confirm the previous baby's death.)
- *24 weeks:* Suggest fetal kick chart for reassurance.
- *28 weeks:* Suggest the couple hire a doppler and teach them to use it.
- *32 weeks:* Suggest the couple write a birth plan.
- *36 weeks:* Discuss the mode of delivery.
- *38 weeks:* Offer CTG for reassurance.

Birth plan

> *I wrote a birth plan to help me express how I was really feeling. Also I didn't have to worry about saying the same thing over and over again to respective shifts of nurses.*

Many hospitals have a birth plan form which can be given to parents to complete. Headings on such a plan may include:

- Who will be present at the birth?
- How will labour be managed?
- What pain relief options have been considered?
- Which birth positions may be adopted?
- How is the third stage to be managed?
- How is the baby to be handled, e.g. first bath, Konakion, direct room in or nursery?
- What is required postnatally, e.g. length of hospital stay, feeding method (breast or bottle) etc.?

Birth essay

> I have found that the essay provides a window for me, as the care provider, through which I can take a look inside. It allows me the opportunity to screen for potential problems, to individualise my care and to maximise a closer and trusting relationship
>
> (Midwife, personal communication)

A birth essay differs from a birth plan in that it is not a list of do's and don'ts but a free-flowing description about what the birth will mean to the parents, how they are feeling about the process, and what ideas they are thinking about.

Encourage the parents to take time whilst they are writing. Writing their ideas down will help them clarify their thinking about what is important to them, and why. Don't give guidelines for the essay. Their decisions should be based on their own thinking. When they have finished it, schedule a birth essay appointment which should be around twice the usual appointment time to enable you to go over the essay and discuss it, point by point.

The essay allows midwives to see if there is anything specific to focus on before, during or after labour. It enables us to individualise our care.

Couples who are particularly anxious during subsequent pregnancy may find it helpful to do two birth essays — a 'pregnancy essay' now to address present feelings and a later 'birth essay' to speak to the birth.

Discussing the plan and/or the essay(s)

It is important to set aside time for full discussion of whatever the parents write. Bereaved couples, more than non-bereaved, know that you can't script birth, but they may still want to script for a living baby. In other words they will do anything in order to try and guarantee a live birth. It is therefore important that you say you cannot guarantee a live birth, although of course you wish you could. Reassure the parents that you will do everything you can to ensure that mother and baby remain alive and healthy whilst maintaining that this outcome is not up to you alone.

At the end of the birth plan appointment thank the couple for taking the time to write. Inform them that their writing will be included with the mother's records, ready for the birth.

Intrapartum

> *I felt confused.*
> *I felt scared and I started to cry.*
> *I felt extremely tense.*
> *I was terrified.*
> *A strange feeling came over me. I felt distant.*
> *I was absolutely beside myself.*
> *I felt like my heart was going to jump out of my mouth it was beating so hard.*

These are quotes from women telling me how they felt whilst they were in labour with a subsequent baby. Although I believe a certain level of fear is almost universal amongst labouring women I think that the depth of fear exuding from the comments above is unusual.

Several women also reported to me feelings of confusion, distance or numbness. I have interpreted these as a form of disorientation, probably brought about by the imminent delivery of another baby triggering memories or even flashbacks to their previous loss.

When you are working with women delivering a subsequent baby after the death of a baby you need to be aware of the previous loss and be sensitive to the anxieties and intrusive flashbacks that subsequent labour may bring. Things that might trigger a flashback in labour are:
- the same or a similar room
- the same or a similar-looking doctor or midwife
- the colour of the walls

- loss of contact or decelerations on the fetal monitor
- positions for pushing
- the act of pushing (since pushing may have meant death last time)
- feelings during delivery.

How you can help

- Acknowledge the previous loss. If the parents are comfortable, ask what the dead baby's name was. Ask if they have named this baby, and if they would like you to use the new baby's name during labour.
- Keep them in the present. Remind them constantly that this is a different labour and a different baby.
- Explain every procedure and give concrete reasons why you know the baby is safe.
- Get support from your co-workers so that the team's workload can be adjusted to allow the couple to have the same carer, as far as possible, for the whole time.
- The father is usually as afraid as the mother. His fear may manifest as anger or questioning of the care you are giving, but he needs just as much support as she does.
- Validate their right to feel anything they feel. Even if they have had support in working with their fears and anxieties, usually they will not act like a 'normal' labouring couple. Their last experience was tragic. They have a right to more care and closer monitoring.

Postpartum

> I have often said that Edward left a round hole in my heart. Although Samantha's birth helped to fill that hole she is a different person and is therefore a different shape and so she only partially fills it. She is a square peg in a round hole. (Warland and Warland, 1996)

Until they get to the postpartum period families do not usually expect it to be difficult. This may be especially true for families whose loss was a few years ago. When the subsequent pregnancy brings the first live birth, sometimes it is not until the new baby comes that parents really realise what they missed with their baby who died.

Many midwives might think that once the parents have a live, healthy baby in their arms they no longer have cause to worry. However, the parents may still be dealing with reminders and pain that simply don't go away. I wrote a poem entitled 'It still hurts' which may help you to see the kind of issues that subsequent parents often face after the birth of the next baby.

It still hurts

You may think, my friend, all is well now I have a live healthy baby in my arms, but it still hurts when I am reminded of my baby who died.

I am reminded when:

She is awake and I see those lovely eyes and I remember how I longed to see those other eyes, now closed forever;

She is asleep and I see my dead baby lying there and I check to see she is still alive;

When I am full of milk waiting for her to wake,

I remember breasts full of milk which I couldn't give to another;

When I bath, change and dress her,

I remember how different it was bathing and dressing her sister for her coffin;

When I am woken at night,
I remember those sleepless nights of grief.

So you see now I have this lovely, precious, live baby
I am constantly reminded of her dead sister.
You expect me to be happy, and so I am,
but it is not a carefree, naïve happiness,
but rather a muted happiness still tinged with sorrow.

(Warland and Warland, 1996)

You can help

How does a midwife help these parents in the postpartum period?

- Acknowledge the baby who died by saying something like 'This must be a bittersweet time for you.'

- Ask if the parents have a photo of the last baby. Ask to see it and comment on any family resemblance or indeed that the babies are not alike.
- Recognise that the parents might call their living baby by their dead baby's name. Reassure the parents that this is common for all parents, not just the bereaved, to call a new baby by a sibling's name.
- Realise that the mother may be a little more likely to experience breastfeeding problems, especially those commonly associated with anxiety.
- Understand that the parents might have an 'unusual' bonding response. Some parents experience great difficulty 'letting go' of their new baby. One mother described feelings of anxiety when anyone cuddled her baby and panic if anyone, including nursing staff, walked out of sight with her baby. Other parents have described a sense of coolness towards their baby — this may be associated with not wanting to 'bond' lest the baby die and grief encompass them once again.
- Notice anniversary times. It may be that the parents are in hospital around the time of the last baby's birth, death, due date, funeral etc. Bereaved parents usually appreciate such times being noted. Simply asking how the parents are feeling can show that you care and remember.
- Help with visitors. The birth of a baby often brings a deluge of visitors. The birth of a living baby after the death of a baby seems to bring all kinds of extra visitors. This flood of people may come just as the couple are feeling exhausted from a long pregnancy and an emotional labour and delivery. Offer your assistance by discussing strategies for managing visitors with the parents.
- Acknowledge fear. If the baby requires care in a nursery the parents are likely to be most anxious. You can assist them by acknowledging their fear, by reassuring them that you expect them to be afraid. Make what allowances you can to accommodate their needs. For example, one mother negotiated for triple bank phototherapy (usually requiring nursery admission) to be carried out in her room.
- Organise an apnoea monitor prior to discharge for those parents who feel the need for that extra assurance.

Conclusion

The midwife's role in a subsequent pregnancy and during subsequent parenting is to:
- help bereaved parents recognise and affirm that their fears and anxieties are normal
- support them in attaching to their new baby
- allow them to continue to love and grieve for the baby who died.

REFERENCES

Crowther ME (1995): Perinatal death: worse obstetric and neonatal outcome in a subsequent pregnancy. *J R Army Med. Corps* 141 (2) June: 92-97.

Katz Rothman B (1988): *The Tentative Pregnancy.* London: Pandora Press.

SAFDA (1995): *Diagnosis of Abnormality in an Unborn Baby. The Impact, Options and Afterwards.* Sydney: NSW Genetics Education Program.

Warland J, Warland M (1996): *Pregnancy after Loss.* Adelaide: Warland.

INTERESTING RESEARCH ARTICLES

Agterberg G et al. (1997): Mothers' trait anxiety and adaptation to an infant born subsequent to the loss of a late pregnancy. *Psychol Rep* 80 (1) Feb.: 216-218.

Armstrong D, Hutti M (1998): Pregnancy after prenatal loss: the relationship between anxiety and prenatal attachment. *Journal of Obstetrics, Gynaecologic and Neonatal Nursing* 10: 183-189.

Cuisiner M et al. (1996): Pregnancy following miscarriage: course of grief and some determining factors. *J Psychosom. Obstet. Gynecol* 17: 168-174.

Davis DL et al. (1989): Postponing pregnancy after perinatal death: perspectives on doctor advice. *J Am Acad Child Adolesc Psychiatry* 28 (4) July: 481-7.

Goldenberg RL et al. (1993): Pregnancy outcome following a second-trimester loss. *Obstet Gynecol* 81 (3) Mar.: 444-446.

Hunfeld JAM et al. (1996): Quality of life and anxiety in pregnancies after late pregnancy loss: A case-control study. *Prenatal Diagnosis* 16: 783-790.

Hunfeld JAM et al. (1997): Trait anxiety, negative emotions, and the mother's adaptation to an infant born subsequent to late pregnancy loss: a case-control study. *Prenatal Diagnosis* 17 (9) Sep.: 843-851.

Mandell F, Wolfe LC (1975): Sudden infant death syndrome and subsequent pregnancy. *Pediatrics* 56 (5) Nov.: 774-776.

O'Leary JM, Thorwick C (1993): Parenting during pregnancy: The infant as the vehicle for intervention in high risk pregnancy. *Int J Prenatal Perinatal Psych Med* 5 (3): 303-310.

Paz JE et al. (1992): Previous miscarriage and stillbirth as risk factors for other unfavorable outcomes in the next pregnancy. *Br Journal Obstet-Gyaecol* 99 (10) Oct.: 808–12.

Peterson G (1994): Chains of grief: The impact of prenatal loss on subsequent pregnancy. *Pre and Perinatal Psychology Journal* 8 (1) Fall.

Phipps S (1985–86): The subsequent pregnancy after stillbirth: anticipatory parenthood in the face of uncertainty. *Int. J. Psychiatry in Medicine* 15 (3).

Stirrat GM (1990): Recurrent miscarriage. *Lancet* 336: 673–675.

Timbers KA, Feinberg RF (1996): Recurrent pregnancy loss: a review. *Nurse-Pract-Forum* 7 (2) June: 64–75.

Theut S et al. (1992) Perinatal loss and maternal attitudes toward the subsequent child. *Infant Ment Health J* 13: 157–166.

Wilson AL et al. (1988): The next baby: parents' responses to perinatal experiences subsequent to a stillbirth. *J Perinatol* 8 Summer, 3: 188–92.

RECOMMENDED READING

Cohen M (1986): *The Shadow of an Angel — diary of a subsequent pregnancy following a neonatal loss.* Los Colinas: Liberal Press.

Davis, Deborah L (1996): *Empty Cradle, Broken Heart: Surviving the Death of Your Baby* 2nd edn. Golden, CO: Fulcrum Publishing.

Ilse S, Doerr M (1996): *Another Baby? Maybe . . .* Maple Plain: Wintergreen Press.

O'Leary J, Parker L, Thorwick C (1998): *After Loss: Parenting in the Next Pregnancy. A manual for professionals working with families in pregnancy following loss.* Minneapolis: Allina Health System.

Pregnancy After A Loss (1993): Minneapolis, MN: Abbott Northwestern Parent Education Program.

Schwibert P, Kirk P (1993): *Still To Be Born.* Portland: Perinatal Loss.

LOOKING AFTER YOURSELF

As for death one gets used to it, even if it's only other people's death you get used to.

(Enid Bagnold)

Caring for bereaved parents is emotionally draining. Health professionals often like to be in control and are usually in a position to be able to make things better. Midwives are especially used to being involved in the happy and the fulfilled. There is no doubt that you can feel vulnerable, helpless, inadequate and overwhelmed by the pain you see in fellow human beings, pain you have no hope of removing from them.

The death of a baby always affects us deeply, perhaps even causing us to question the purpose and meaning of life. It may affect us personally, especially if we have children or babies of our own. It may cause us to be grateful for, and perhaps even fearful for, our own children's lives.

However, for all the emotional drain that caring for bereaved families can engender it can also be very rewarding, both personally and professionally. Knowing you have done your best to make a difference for a family, knowing that they will remember you and the impact that you have had on their lives may seem incredible to you but it is true.

There is no doubt that caring for someone whose baby dies is a critical incident for you. For many years, routine debriefing after a critical incident was not offered to staff in hospitals. Probably that is still the case in some hospitals. Many staff seem to try to get by with chatting informally over a cup of coffee. However, it is very important to resolve the effect of the incident in a structured as well as an informal way. We need to acknowledge and talk about our fears and anxieties by way of formal debriefing.

I completed my nursing training in an era when it was certainly considered to be unprofessional to be seen shedding tears at work. Many of my colleagues would still feel this to be unprofessional behaviour. However, I have heard over and over again at support meetings for bereaved parents just how much those parents really valued the tears of the health professionals who cared for them. They saw this as sharing their pain. I believe that it is perfectly appropriate to cry with the family. Furthermore, if you are not the type who cries easily, it is very important to tell bereaved parents that you 'feel' for them or indicate how sorry you are simply by saying 'I'm sorry your baby died'. Otherwise parents may believe you to be cold hearted.

> Those of us who have suffered perinatal losses in years gone by are sometimes broadsided by a brief poignant moment, and the resultant tears are tears for ourselves and our own lost children. Other times, the utter helplessness seems unbearable. And those unanswerable questions, those 'whys' and 'what ifs', can remind us of our own struggles with the mysteries of our faith. (Frizell, 1997)

These are not moments to hide from newly bereaved parents; rather, they provide a starting point in empathy from which bereaved parents can usually benefit.

Unburdening yourself to your spouse/partner, mother, father, or other family and friends may be well and good, however you tend not to be able to do that for very long before they either become tired of hearing it or simply don't understand. It is important that you find some kind of structured peer support either through a hospital counsellor or some other trained listener, someone who can listen to you and with whom you can debrief. This person needs to be someone whom you can trust to listen to you and to keep confidential any information that you may reveal

BURNOUT

Apart from debriefing after caring for a bereaved family, midwives, like many other workers, need to look after themselves at work generally in order to avoid burnout. Burnout is a syndrome of emotional exhaustion, depersonalisation, and reduced personal accomplishment that can occur among individuals who do 'people work' of some kind. It is a response to the chronic emotional strain of dealing extensively with human beings, particularly when they are troubled or are having problems. Burnout is one type of response to job stress. Although it has some of the same deleterious effects as other stress responses, what is unique about burnout is that the stress arises from the social interaction between helper and recipient.

Preventing burnout

- Be aware that caring for bereaved parents is emotionally draining.
- Avoid moving, in the same shift, between care of women who have suffered a stillbirth and those anticipating a live birth.
- Avoid being alone when handling a dead baby. Have either a parent or a colleague with you.
- You must be comfortable when you are providing care, so avoid looking after families if you have deep personal or religious objections to some aspect of their care. You should not be made to feel guilty but neither should they.
- Be aware of and learn to use the knowledge and back-up of those around you.
- Avoid always allocating the same person to care for bereaved parents — that can almost guarantee burnout. While that one person may do a wonderful job, others need to care for these families too. The most experienced person can be the resource/back-up person for all the midwives on the team.
- Always communicate with your peers.

When you are actually caring for families it will be helpful if you can accept that you:
- don't know everything and are not *usually* personally responsible when bad things happen
- don't know all the answers and don't expect to provide parents with the answers
- don't always know what to say — silence is often the best response
- will be helpful to some but not to others
- need the help of your colleagues
- are not perfect
- have strengths you can draw on and weaknesses to overcome
- can be open about expressing your feelings
- cannot be all things to all people all of the time
- can say no when extra commitments will cause pressure.

Activities to help you avoid burnout

- Schedule regular 'me-time' for activities you enjoy, e.g. relaxing in a deep bath, reading a book, walking along the beach.
- Develop a support network of peers, people that you trust who may be working in a field similar to your own who can contact you if they have had a bad day and who will welcome similar contact from you.
- If you care for bereaved families often you should organise a regular debriefing with a trained counsellor.
- Surround yourself with growing things — plants, pets — that will provide an interest as well as stress relief.
- Take short breaks regularly from your job.
- Let off steam with a very physical activity.
- Institute amongst your workmates the practice of giving regular 'warm fuzzies'. (At the finish of a course I did once participants were invited to give each other a 'warm fuzzy'. Each person wrote something complimentary on a piece of paper about each other member of the group and then gave it to its intended recipient. I ended up with 15 'warm fuzzies' which still warm my heart when I read them.)
- Establish for yourself interests that have nothing to do with work.
- Prioritise your life's activities in order to avoid being 'snowed under'.
- Eat regular meals.
- Take regular exercise.
- Develop regular, solid sleep habits.
- Build up a PMA (positive mental attitude).
- Learn to recognise when a situation is causing you stress and work out quickly how to deal with it.
- Be gentle on yourself.

To avert stress it is important we recognise our own signs and symptoms of stress. Also we need to be aware of what increases our stress and how we can relieve it.

Stress

Ways to increase stress
- Bottle up your feelings.
- Place high or unrealistic expectations on yourself.
- Think too far into the future.

Ways to decrease stress
- Value and foster the good relationships you have.
- Enjoy the good things in life.
- Find the humour that is in every situation.

Finally it is important to realise that you are a physical, mental, emotional, spiritual, and relational being with a need to look after every aspect of your life in order to remain healthy.

REFERENCES

Bagnold, Edith (1889–1981), British novelist, playwright, *Autobiography* (1969): ch. 16. As quoted in *The Columbia Dictionary of Quotations* (1993) licensed from Columbia University Press.

Frizell Judy (1997): Untitled. *MEND Newsletter* 2 (4) July/August.

Vogel G (1996): *A Caregivers Handbook to Perinatal Loss.* St Paul: DeRuyter-Nelson Publications.

INTERESTING RESEARCH ARTICLES

Jenkins S, Wingate C (1994): Who cares for young carers? *BMJ* 308(6931) 19 Mar.: 733–734.

Kelly D (1989): Stress and how to avoid professional burnout. *Midwife, Health Visitor and Community Nurse* 25 (5) May: 172–177

Lewis L (1995): Caring for the carers. *Mod Midwife* 5 (2) Feb.: 7–10.

Syverson C (1997): The young ones. *Nursing Times* 93 (24) 11 June: 28–29.

RECOMMENDED READING

Ilse S (1996) *Giving Care, Taking Care.* Maple Plain, MN: Wintergreen Press.

Maslach C (1986): *Burnout — the Cost of Caring.* Engelwood Cliffs: Prentice Hall Inc.

Vineyard S (1989): *How To Take Care of You ... So You Can Take Care of Others.* Downs Grove: Heritage Arts Publishing.

APPENDIX TWO

MEN

Why is it that no one seems to care about me? Why don't people know that I loved my baby and I hurt like hell that she has died? Do they believe that just because I am a man I do not feel the pain of her death? Men do feel pain. Men do hurt. Men are vulnerable but we are not expected to show it. I just wish that someone would remember that she was my baby too.

(Jones, 1996)

It may be that, in the early stages of grief, men and women both experience shock together. It may be that, at least for this time, their grief 'feels' identical but this is a misapprehension and, as time passes, the different grieving styles of the man and the woman will become increasingly obvious. If the couple do not understand what is going on then there is likely to be some strain on their relationship. Part of the midwife's role is to prepare the couple for differences in their grieving styles so that they will be better equipped to cope with the differences that occur.

Most fathers describe themselves as attached to their baby but not as attached as their female partner (Worth, 1997).

Mothers are often treated as somehow different than fathers. Comments like 'How is your wife?' are very common and often hurtful to men. Harold E. Jones's quote above expresses beautifully the fact that men hurt too. Men do not have moment-by-moment contact with their baby during the pregnancy. Studies have shown that men begin to bond with their baby only once it becomes real to them, either during the 18-week scan or when they can feel fetal movements (Mercer, 1998). Maternal bonding may begin much earlier in the pregnancy than this. However, men may have an opportunity to bond with the baby after its birth, well before the mother does. If the mother has a general anaesthetic for a Caesarean birth then the father may see and hold his baby well before the mother. In some cases he may have sole contact with his dying baby.

Men may not express their grief as openly as women, leading the woman to think he doesn't care about their baby. This may lead to marital tension, especially if the relationship was already strained.

Staudacher (1991) points out the social expectations that are placed on men. Men are expected to be:
- courageous
- sexually potent
- a provider
- in control
- more concerned with thinking than feeling.

When a baby dies it is usually not possible for men to meet any of these social expectations. This inability may result in the man feeling helpless, as Vredevelt (1995) recounts:

> After I found out about our baby's death, I kept wanting to do something to make things better, to change things. But there was nothing I could do to give our baby life again. I couldn't alter our baby's destiny and was frustrated by being so helpless.

MALE BEHAVIOUR

> Most men respond to the death of their baby in the way that they have been taught to behave, are expected to behave and are capable of behaving. (Jones, 1996).

Men who have lost their babies may feel and behave in certain ways.
- They may feel a failure because they think they should always be in control. The death of their baby shatters their world because it is something beyond their control.
- They may hide their emotions because they fear that to openly express how they feel will be considered a weakness and may make them vulnerable to further hurt.
- They sometimes give the impression to their wives and children that they have not been affected by the loss. When the man refuses to show how he really feels, he generally wears a mask that is misinterpreted as his not having been affected by what has happened.
- Many men believe that it is their role to be strong and supportive, to be the one available for other family members to lean on. So when their baby dies they 'tough it out' and act 'strong' for the rest of the family.

Some men 'lock into' what may be described as a 'loving protector' or 'provider/fixer' role which means they act in particular ways:

- They try to delay or stop their own grief reactions ('put their grief on hold') in order to establish control for the sake of the family.
- They fulfil the expectation that men are responsible for solving family problems and helping the family deal with major crises.
- They make decisions for their partners because they believe they are expected to take charge in a crisis situation and be the leader.
- Most men will immediately become the 'loving protector', doing whatever they can to shield their partner and family from further hurt.
- Because many men believe that any outward sign of grief on the part of their partner or family is evidence that they have failed in their loving protector role they discourage their partner from grieving. These men cannot bear any further sign of failure, so they insist that the family 'gets on with life'.(Jones, 1996)

As Jones (1996) reported:

> At times, the father was so busy supporting his wife that his own needs were being neglected.

HOW A MIDWIFE CAN HELP A MAN TO HELP HIS PARTNER AND HIMSELF

- Acknowledge him as a father.
- Expect him to grieve and give him permission to express openly how he is feeling. Provide him with as many opportunities as his partner to parent his dead or dying baby.
- Encourage him to use his child's name in conversation.
- Postpone important decisions such as autopsy and funeral arrangements until both parents are able to make the decision together. Don't expect the man to make these decisions on behalf of his partner.
- Make some time just to sit with him. Don't ignore him.
- Encourage him not to ring everyone they know to pass on the bad news. Suggest he call a few of his close family and friends and ask them to pass on the message to others.
- Ask him to stay with his partner, even if he is feeling helpless and useless, because his presence will be valued

---

- Urge him to reschedule his work commitments so that he can spend more time with his family. After all, if the baby had lived, he would probably have made some adjustments. His presence is required just as much because the baby has died.
- Let him know that men and women grieve differently and at different rates. Tell him that it is important not to expect too much of each other too soon after the baby's death.
- Make him aware that he will need to be patient with his partner as they ride the roller coaster of emotions over the coming months.
- Encourage him to communicate with his partner. 'A problem shared is a problem halved' is very true in this situation.
- Suggest that he take the initiative to plan a dinner out or a holiday. She may not have the emotional energy to plan such an event but will welcome the break it affords them both.
- Ask him to be present at the postnatal visit to share the reliving, to ask questions and to help remember what will be said.
- Warn him that anniversary times may be particularly difficult and encourage him to use his natural 'loving protector' role to shield his family from difficult situations. Baptisms and family birthday celebrations that crop up in the early days of grief are often very painful.
- Encourage him to take control of his family life — surviving children need at least one parent available to them at any given time. Initially he may feel a little more emotionally able to care for children than his partner does.
- Make him aware that his partner was not to blame in any way for their baby's death. Let him know that his partner may well express guilt over what has happened and that when she does he can reassure her she is not to blame.
- Encourage him to express his love and affection for his partner with more hugs, kisses and flowers than may be usual. However, warn him that it may take some time before sexual relations are resumed.
- Help him to understand that men and women grieve differently. What works for him will not work if imposed on her and vice versa.

REFERENCES

Jones Harold E (1996): Male grief. Keynote address presented to SANDS 6th National Conference. Adelaide, October 1996.

Mercer RT et al. (1988): Further exploration of maternal and paternal fetal attachment. *Res Nurs Health* 11 (2) Apr.: 83–95.

Staudacher C (1991): *Men and Grief: A Guide for Men Surviving the Death of a Loved One.* Oakland: New Harbinger.

Vredevelt P (1995): *Empty Arms.* Sisters: Multnomah Press.

Worth N (1997): Becoming a father to a stillborn child. *Clinical Nursing Research* 6 (1) Feb.: 71–89.

INTERESTING RESEARCH ARTICLES

Cordell A, Thomas N (1990): Fathers and grieving: Coping with infant death. *Journal of Perinatology* 10 (1): 75–80.

Miron J, Chapman JS (1994): Supporting men's experiences with the event of their partners' miscarriage. *Can J Nurs-Res* 26 (2) Summer: 61–72.

Revak-Lutz RJ, Kellner KR (1994): Paternal involvement after perinatal death. *J Perinatology* 14 (6) Nov.–Dec.: 442–5.

Zachariah R (1994): Maternal–fetal attachment: influence of mother–daughter and husband–wife relationships. *Res Nurs Health* 17 (1) Feb.: 37–44.

Zlotogorski Z et al. (1997): Parental attitudes toward obstetric ultrasound examination. *J Obstet Gynaecol Res* 23 (1) Feb.: 25–8.

RECOMMENDED READING

Golden Thomas R (1997): *Swallowed by a Snake: The Gift of the Masculine Side of Healing.* Gaithersburg: Golden Healing Pub.

Loizeaux W (1993): *Anna: A Daughter's Life.* New York: Arcade Publishing.

Nelson T (1994): *A Father's Story.* St Paul: A Place to Remember.

Schatz W (1994): *Healing a Father's Grief.* Oak Brook: Compassionate Friends.

Tister M, Torrell S (1991): *Healing Together: For Couples Grieving the Death of Their Baby.* Omaha: Centering Corporation.

Wheat R (1995): *Miscarriage: A Man's Book.* Omaha: Centering Corporation.

CHILDREN AND GRIEF

When my doctor sat me down to tell me that my baby was dead, I immediately asked him how I should explain this to my son. It surprised me when he said he had never had anyone ever ask him that before. He had no suggestions for me at all.

INTRODUCTION

Midwives don't usually tell children directly about the loss of their sibling however it may be that the bereaved couple will ask you for suggestions on how to explain the death of their baby to their surviving child/ren.

A CHILD'S GRIEF

The grief of a child is more complex than that of an adult, for a number of reasons. If a child loses a parent, that parent is lost. A child who loses a sibling loses not only that sibling but also both parents, for a time. A child may find, following the death of a baby, that one parent becomes 'lost' through divorce, because the rate of family breakdown after the death of a baby is high.

Children revisit their grief as they mature. A 10-year old understands and can process much more than a 5-year old. Psychological time is different from chronological time in that when the child is ready there is work to be done. A child who loses a sibling will revisit grief many times before adulthood.

Grief has been likened to an onion — as you peel away the layers it makes you cry. But often children don't show their grief by crying. One child, in talking of her own situation, exhibited behaviour that is common:

> *I don't like to show my emotions. If I cry it makes my mum cry and I don't like it when she cries.*

Children generally want to protect their parents:

> *It's hard to talk to my mum because I hate to see her cry.*

Children will use different media to express their grief. Adults, including midwives, can help children by facilitating different modes of expression — drawing will show what the child's grief looks like; making sounds or songs will show you what it sounds like; movement or dance can show you what the grief feels like. To help a child express grief through drawing, try using a colour wheel. Get the child to draw a colour wheel or pie chart with emotions expressed in different colours. Let the child choose the emotions (e.g. sad, angry, confused, wounded, guilty, ignored, worried, mad, weird, irresponsible, happy), the colours that depict those emotions, the percentage of each colour that the emotion arouses and the amount of 'space' on the colour wheel that each emotion takes up. This activity can give the parents an idea of how children are feeling. If the activity is repeated after some time has passed, it will be possible to see how the children are progressing in their own grief.

Children don't understand the difference between what they feel and what they know so they can feel abandoned. One child expressed this vulnerability by saying:

> *Children aren't very protected.*

Parents may be tempted to shield their surviving children from the trauma of seeing their dead sibling but it is very important that this is not done. Children are being taught constantly how to respond to the world and life events by the way adults around them respond to these events. If children are shielded from this life event then they will be poorer for missing the experience. This experience will have an impact on them whether they are shielded from it or not. Children are intuitive beings and may be very well aware of what is going on. The baby cannot simply disappear just because he has died. Something must be said to the children. Children have a way of finding out if they have been lied to, even years after an event, and therefore it is wise to tell the truth.

You should encourage parents to allow their children to come to the hospital to see their dead sibling. Surviving children need to feel that the baby is a part of their family. When a baby sibling dies, parents and children need lots of hugs. Living children can be such a comfort.

EXPLAINING THE DEATH

A good rule of thumb is to keep explanations simple and clear. Parents may need guidance from you about what to say. Following are some examples of 'explanations' that parents might use to explain to their children what has happened to their baby:

- 'The baby was not strong like you and she died.'
- 'The baby was too little and he died.'
- 'We don't know why the baby died but we do know that you are too big to die the way the baby did.'

WHAT NOT TO SAY TO CHILDREN

- Avoid referring to the baby as 'lost'. Young children lose things all the time and find them again.
- Avoid saying 'God has taken the baby' because children might think they will be the next to be taken.
- Don't imply that the baby was too good to live. The surviving sibling might think they have to be bad or they will die too.
- Don't say the baby 'got sick and died' because children may fear that they too will die the next time they become ill.
- Refrain from implying that the baby is 'sleeping' as a child may then become fearful of dying whilst asleep.
- Refrain from trying to answer questions a child has not asked. Children are well able to ask questions if they want more information.

SAYING GOODBYE

Parents may ask midwives if their children will be okay to go to the funeral. Reassure them that including the children is usually beneficial to both the child and the family, as this parent found:

> *I didn't want to distress my youngest child and wondered whether to take her to the funeral. We did take her and we are now very glad that we did because she remembers being there and remembers putting flowers on the coffin. I believe we would regret it now if we hadn't taken her.*

> *It was great having children at the funeral. They lightened the
> atmosphere a lot. Some played hopscotch on the graves and
> one of the little ones almost fell into our baby's open grave.
> Having children there seemed to make the funeral very
> normal and natural.*

Children can help plan a funeral by:
- making a picture book about the baby
- giving something to the baby at the funeral — a flower on the coffin, a stuffed toy etc.
- reading a suitable book (see recommended reading list) and making suggestions from it
- choosing something for the funeral, e.g. a favourite song, story or poem.

HOW MIDWIVES CAN HELP BEREAVED PARENTS TO HELP THEIR CHILDREN

- Encourage the parents not to hide their tears from their children. If a happy event occurred children would not be shielded from seeing their parents laugh so the children should not be shielded from their parents' tears. If children are exposed to adults crying at sad times they will learn a valuable lesson, namely, that it's okay to cry at times of sadness.
- Suggest the parents use this experience to teach their child/ren about death as an inevitable part of life.
- Tell the parents to reassure their child/ren that their baby's death was no-one's fault. Many children have 'magical thinking' and imagine they are somehow responsible for the baby's death.
- Inform parents that their child may not be able to tell them in terms other than by their behaviour how they are feeling, e.g. when a child is tired he may not be able to tell you he wishes to go to bed but you can tell from his behaviour that he needs to go. Likewise a change in behaviour may indicate the child's nonverbal need for reassurance. Warn parents to expect their child/ren may act differently in the next few weeks and months and that such behaviour is most likely linked to the baby's death until proven otherwise.

- Urge the parents to be lavish with their affection. Many children will feel confused or upset. Parents may be unaware of the adverse effect their grief state is having on their child/ren. They can offer a great deal of reassurance by hugging and kissing their child/ren a little more than usual.
- Let the parents know that it is okay to seek outside help in the form of family therapy if they feel that they or their child/ren are having difficulty coping with the loss.
- Reassure the parents that their children will be okay.

The couple are likely to find their children a benefit and a disadvantage at the same time. Many bereaved parents are grateful that they have a living child or children and yet they have a constant visual and (probably) noisy reminder that there was a sibling who died. Bereaved parents who have young children should be encouraged to try to plan some time together away from the children every week to release built-up stress.

GENETIC TERMINATION

When a pregnancy is terminated for genetic reasons other children may well be aware of something being wrong. The parents need to decide together what to tell the children and they may ask for suggestions from you about what to tell their children. Remind them that, depending on the age of the child/ren, they may need reassurance that nothing bad is going to happen to them. Children must also be reassured that they are not to blame. One family said:

> *We chose to inform our children that the baby was not strong or healthy.*

INTERESTING RESEARCH ARTICLES

Birenbaum L et al. (1990): The response of children to the dying and death of a sibling. *Omega Journal of Death and Dying* 20 (3): 213-228.

Bray C (1981): Children's grief after a cot death. *Aust Soc Work* 34 (2): 31-37.

Davies B (1993): Sibling bereavement: research-based guidelines for nurses. *Seminars in Oncology Nursing* 9 (2): 107–113.

Davies B (1994): Behind youthful masks — the experience of sibling bereavement. Paper presented to the conference of the National Association of Loss and Grief. Adelaide, September.

Kranzler E et al. (1990): Early childhood bereavement. *Journal of American Academy of Child and Adolescent Psychiatry* 29 (4): 513–519.

O'Toole M et al. (1995): Creative interventions with bereaved siblings. Paper presented to Association for Welfare of Children Conference. Melbourne.

Siegel K (1990): A Prevention Program for Bereaved Children. *American Journal of Orthopsychiatry* 60 (2): 168–175.

Williams ML (1995): Sibling reaction to cot death. *The Medical Journal of Australia* 5 Sept.: 227–231.

RECOMMENDED READING FOR CHILDREN

Bryte M (1988): *No New Baby.* Omaha: Centering Corporation.
This book is for children whose expected sibling dies in early-to-mid-pregnancy.

Cohn J (1995): *Molly's Rosebud.* Morton Grove: Albert Whitman Co.
Written for children on the topic of miscarriage, the story is told in a straightforward manner and openly examines the fears that might confront siblings after a miscarriage.

Crouthamel T (1986): *It's OK.* Langeloth: Keystone Press.
Written by a bereaved father to help his son and other children cope with the death of a sibling, this book is a survival kit for bereaved siblings.

Dodge N (1984): *Thumpy's Story: The story of grief and loss shared by Thumpy the bunny.* Springfield: Prairie Lark Press.
Thumpy's sister dies suddenly because she is not strong enough to live.

Erling J (1994): *Our Baby Died. Why?* St Paul: A Place To Remember.
Jake, who is 7 years old, tells the story of his dreams for a new brother and his devastation when Jesse is stillborn. Jake shares his grief from a child's perspective and relates the story of a subsequent pregnancy and birth of his twin siblings.

Murray J (1993): 'An Ache in Their Hearts' Resource Package. Brisbane: The University of Queensland.
The kit includes several books for children.

Grollman A (1993): *Straight Talk about Death for Teenagers.* Boston: Beacon Press.
The book explains likely grief reactions, the effect of grief on relationships and how to deal with funerals.

Goldstein Rand J (no date): *Where's Jess?* Omaha: Centering Corporation.
This is the story of a cot death baby.

Klein N (1974): *Confessions of an Only Child.* New York: Pantheon Books.
Antonia, who is 9 years old, anticipates the birth of a new sibling who dies.

Old W (1995): *Stacy Had a Little Sister.* Morton Grove: Albert Whitman Company.
The book speaks to the issues and concerns of many siblings who have lost a baby brother or sister.

Scrivani Mark (1991): *When Death Walks In.* Omaha: Centering Corporation.
This book for teenagers deals with specific aspects of the grieving process.

Stickney D (1974): *Waterbugs and Dragonflies.* London: Mowbray.
In simple terms this story explains the permanence and irreversibility of death.

Warland J (1994): *Our Baby Died.* Melbourne: Joint Board of Christian Education.
Told from a child's perspective, this is the story of what happens in a family when a baby is stillborn.

Weir A (1992): *Am I Still a Big Sister?* Newton: Fallen Leaf Press.
Elisabeth Kübler-Ross calls this 'a wonderful book for siblings who have lost a brother or sister.'

RECOMMENDED READING FOR ADULTS

Dyregov A (1991): *Grief in Children.* London: Jessica Kingsley.

Fitzgerald H (1992): *The Grieving Child.* Omaha: Centering Corporation.

Goldman L (1994): *Life & Loss: A Guide to Helping Grieving Children.* Muncie: Accelerated Development.

La Tour K (1991): *For Those Who Live: Helping Children Cope with the Loss of a Brother or Sister.* Omaha: Centering Corporation.

Levy E (1982): *Children Are Not Paper Dolls.* Springfield: Human Service Press.

Morgan J (1991): *Young People and Death.* Philadelphia: The Charles Press Publishers.

Rosen H (1986): *Unspoken Grief: Coping with Childhood Sibling Loss.* New York: Lexington Books.

Schaefer D, Lyons C (1993): *How Do We Tell the Children? Helping children understand and cope with separation and loss.* New York: Newmarket Press.

Webb Nancy (1993): *Helping Bereaved Children.* New York: The Guilford Press.

GRANDPARENTS

So often the forgotten mourners, grandparents frequently experience something of a 'double whammy' when their grandchild dies. They not only lose their grandchild, who represents the family's hope for the future and the continuation of the family, but also they have to watch helplessly as their child suffers terrible pain. Not only that, they will see over time that their child will never be the same again. This can be quite upsetting for someone of the older generation to witness.

Many times the grandparents may be from an era when a baby who died was not seen, or held and never mentioned in the family. They may therefore be appalled at current midwifery practice. Your job is to encourage them to participate in their children's memory creation. Include them in photos and reassure them that it is acceptable to cuddle their grandchild and say their goodbyes.

HOW MIDWIVES CAN HELP GRANDPARENTS TO HELP THEIR CHILD

- Tell them that there is no way they can take away their child's pain; this is not something you can kiss better.
- Help them to see that grief is not something they can take on for their child instead of their child. Grief is a 'do it yourself' job.
- Make them aware that they can be supportive but should not be overprotective.
- Help them to realise that they can do what their child needs them to do.

- Tell them they need to ask their child's permission before they do anything that may have consequences on grief recovery, e.g. some grandparents dismantle the nursery in the mistaken belief that this would be a distressing activity for their child.
- Encourage them to participate in family photos and then to display the photo as they would a photo of a living grandchild.
- Warn them that they may revisit losses from their own lives, especially if they had a baby who died.
- Help them to realise that they must not feel guilty for the grandchild dying, even if the reason for the baby's death is any kind of genetic predisposition. Many grandparents will question the cause and some may place the blame on their child's in-law family, declaring that 'nothing like this has ever happened on our side of the family before'.
- Support and understand them if they experience what could be described best as survivor guilt, feeling guilty that they are still alive when a baby has died. Many grandparents wish they could have died in place of the baby. Even though this is not possible it is still a real and sincere wish of many bereaved grandparents.
- Help them if they need to talk about their dead grandchild but feel unable to talk with their child lest they upset them. Introduce them to organisations such as SANDS or other community support groups, just as you will have introduced the parents.
- Tell them that they may be able to help themselves by helping their child in a practical way — cooking a meal, doing some ironing, or looking after surviving children. Grief is an energy-sapping experience and some bereaved parents find that they don't have the energy to be able to offer their children the kind of practical support that they might need.
- Urge them to keep open the lines of communication. When family members are honest about how they feel, confusion is minimised.
- Warn them to watch for physical signs of grief — stomach pain, diarrhoea, general aches and pains, even chest pain.

RECOMMENDED READING

Gerner M (1990): *For Bereaved Grandparents.* Omaha: Centering Corporation. *This book was written by a bereaved mother and grandmother specifically to help grandparents address their feelings following the death of a grandchild.*

Ilse S, Leininger L (1994): *Grieving Grandparents.* St Paul: Wintergreen Press. *This booklet discusses feelings and situations frequently experienced by grandparents who have lost a grandchild because of miscarriage, stillbirth, or infant death. Topics include communicating feelings, creating memories of the grandchild, 'saying goodbye', reacting to the death, coping, and helping the parents through the experience. A discussion of subsequent pregnancy includes suggestions for how grandparents can lend support.*

Vander Meyden, C (1994): *When Joy Withers Away.* St Paul: A Place to Remember. *A grandfather of a SIDS victim tells his story and gives his suggestions about how grandparents can deal with such a tragedy.*

CULTURAL/RELIGIOUS CONSIDERATIONS

Everything we do, every decision we make and course of action we take is based on our consciously and unconsciously chosen beliefs, attitudes and values.

(Uustal, 1997)

There is no doubt that, many times, the death of a baby causes people to turn to their religious belief and cultural traditions to help them cope with and express their grief. In this brief appendix, it is impossible to cover every belief and every custom in every culture. However, we need to understand that families have different needs and grief cycles based on their cultural, social and personal differences.

Parents themselves will be well aware of their cultural needs and, if asked, will be able to tell midwives working with them what those needs are. If there is a language barrier it is essential to obtain the services of a translator to ensure that all religious and cultural rites are carried out in accordance with the parents' wishes. If you find yourself in this situation, you may need to contact interpreters and community workers to ensure that the cultural needs of the couple are considered and met.

AT OR AROUND DEATH

Many cultures have important religious rites to be observed at or around the time of death. These may include baptism, blessing or 'last rites'. Usually an ordained minister of the religion will attend to perform the rite.

It is absolutely crucial that midwives do not attempt to perform any religious rite without the express permission of the parents. In one situation I know of, a midwife baptised a baby who was deteriorating rapidly. When the parents were told of this action they were distraught. Their religious denomination opposed infant baptism. They then had not only to grieve for their dead baby but also to come to terms with a baptism that should not have occurred.

Some religions have strict rules as to who may touch a dead body. Asking family members if there are any such restrictions before you act is preferable to trying to rectify a misunderstanding after the event.

Autopsy

Adherents of some religions are forbidden to agree to an autopsy. In other cases an autopsy can be performed but it must be according to strict guidelines about what goes on during and after the autopsy.

Interment

Some faiths require that the interment occurs quickly after the death. This may limit the parents' opportunities for contact with their baby. If you are caring for someone whose religion incorporates these beliefs, be creative about how you facilitate parenting after the baby's death.

AUSTRALIAN ABORIGINES

There are over 250 distinct Australian Aboriginal tribes with their own languages and traditions. Most tribal Aboriginal people will feel uncomfortable in a Western hospital setting. You will need to ask them how best you can meet their needs in the situation in which you find yourselves. Finding an appropriate Aboriginal intermediary may be a good option.

VIETNAMESE

The Vietnamese family often place complete faith in the actions of their caregivers. If a baby was born or became seriously ill, any action directed at helping the child is usually acceptable. The parents will adopt a compliant and deferential relationship with their caregivers. They may be reluctant to ask questions because they completely trust the actions of people caring for their baby. If ongoing care or medication is required, it is important that the baby's grandmother be instructed as she will have a major role in the child's care.

If the baby dies at birth or is stillborn it is most common that the parents will refuse to see it initially. It may be preferred if the baby is wrapped and taken quietly from the room.

The grieving period and parental wishes for the care of their child (i.e. photographs, mementoes, contact etc.) will be influenced by the family structure, their links with a religion and the circumstances relating to the death of the baby. (Dugard, 1989)

The following list outlines some religious beliefs and likely practices associated with them.

BAHA'I

Baptism: No rite.
Death: The local Baha'i community should be contacted to make arrangements in conjunction with the deceased family.
Photos: Acceptable
Autopsy: If required by law
Interment: Embalming is discouraged. The body is buried in a cotton or silk shroud within one hour's journey of the place of death.

BUDDHIST

Baptism: No rite.
Death: Calmness at time of death is considered important. Think about moving the baby to a quiet room away from monitors and noise. Parents may pray, meditate and think virtuous thoughts to assist the baby to a good rebirth. Great importance is attributed to a clear state of mind at the time of death. Therefore, if sedative drugs are being administered, the preferences of the parents need to be determined.
Photos: Acceptable. Photos will assist the parents to focus on the baby as they pray for a good rebirth.
Autopsy: Only after 3–7 days, once the 'inner breath' has ceased.
Interment: In Tibet bodies are 'given' to the birds. In Western culture cremation is common. Burial will occur if the baby has died from a contagious disease.

CHURCH OF JESUS CHRIST OF LATTER DAY SAINTS (MORMON)

Baptism: No infant baptism whilst the baby is living but baptism of the dead is essential; a living person may serve as proxy.
Death: The gospel is preached to the dead.
Photos: Acceptable.
Autopsy: Usually acceptable.
Interment: Cremation is discouraged.

EASTERN ORTHODOX

Baptism: Infant baptism by total immersion followed immediately by confirmation.
Death: 'Last rites' are administered.
Photos: Acceptable.
Autopsy: Acceptable.
Interment: Burial is favoured.

GREEK ORTHODOX

Baptism: Baptism is extremely important but is only for the living. If the baby is gravely ill a priest should be called a soon as possible. In extremis, if it is not possible to baptise by water, the church allows an orthodox lay person to baptise 'in the air' by lifting the baby three times in the name of the Father, Son and Holy Spirit.
Death: No essential ritual.
Photos: According to the family's wishes.
Autopsy: Acceptable.
Interment: No formal funeral is required for 'sinless' children under the age of 3. The baby may be buried with a simple ceremony. No cremation.

HINDU

Baptism: No rite.

Death: The dying baby is placed with his head facing east. A member of the baby's family will chant a sacred chant in the baby's right ear. Immediately after death holy water will be poured into the baby's mouth and the family will wash the body. They are particular about who touches the body. A priest may tie a thread around the neck or wrist to signify blessing. The thread should not be removed.

Photos: Acceptable but only with consent.

Interment: Bodies must be cremated before the sun sets.

JUDAISM

Baptism: No rite but ritual circumcision of boys on the 8th day of life.

Death: During the last minutes of life it is customary that no-one leave the room, out of respect to the dying person. After death the eyes must be closed and the body covered. The feet must point towards the doorway. Parents and other close relatives may rend their clothes to express their grief. It is preferred that non-Jewish people handle the baby as little as possible. There will be ritual washing at the funeral parlour by a group of Jewish people. Orthodox Jews will stay with the baby from death until burial.

Photos: Acceptable.

Autopsy: All Orthodox Jews are opposed

Interment: Burial should take place as soon as possible (within 24 hours) unless it involves the Sabbath (Saturday), then it will be delayed. Burial may also be delayed in order to allow relatives who live a distance away, time to attend. Cremation is absolutely forbidden. It is preferable to bury rather than discard a fetus.

ISLAM

Baptism: No baptism

Death: Verses may be recited from the Quran as the baby is dying. If the baby dies before its first bath it is helpful to ask the parents if they would like to bath the baby. At the funeral parlour the family follow a specified procedure for washing and shrouding the dead.

Photos: Usually acceptable but obtain consent.

Autopsy: No autopsy unless required by law; no body part should be removed.

Interment:The soul enters the fetus after quickening and is thereafter accorded all rites of passage. No rites are required before quickening.The baby is shrouded in white and buried facing Mecca, in an unmarked grave without a coffin. Muslims require burial as soon as possible, ideally within 24 hours. No cremation.

PROTESTANT

(including Anglican, Assemblies of God, Baptist, Lutheran, Uniting, Pentecostal, Presbyterian, Salvation Army)

Baptism: Some are opposed to infant baptism, others will baptise the baby, some may dedicate the dead baby.

Death: Some may anoint the sick or dying baby.

Photos:Acceptable

Autopsy:Acceptable

Interment: Either burial or cremation.

ROMAN CATHOLIC

Baptism: Infant baptism is important and urgent if the infant's prognosis is poor. Any person may use 'emergency' baptism if a priest cannot be called in time. (You baptise by pouring water over the top of the baby's head in the name of the Father, the Son and the Holy Spirit.) A dead baby may not be baptised but it may be blessed and named.

Death:A baptised baby may be anointed. 'Last rites' are performed — prayers for the dying.

Photos:Acceptable.

Autopsy:Acceptable.

Interment:According to the parents' preference.Traditional Roman Catholic families will prefer burial.

RUSSIAN ORTHODOX

Baptism: Only by a priest and only on certain days.

Death:The arms must be placed so that the index fingers form a cross. Clothing must be of a natural fibre so the body will disintegrate into dust as quickly as possible.

Photos: Acceptable.

Autopsy: Not acceptable.

Interment: No embalming or cremation.

SEVENTH DAY ADVENTIST

Baptism: No infant baptism.

Death:The pastor will anoint a dead or dying baby in the name of the Lord.

Photos:Acceptable.

Autopsy: Acceptable.

Interment: Either cremation or burial.

REFERENCES

Dugard L (1989): *Multicultural Information for Midwives*. Canberra: ACMI.

Uustal D (1997): Values-based leadership: character counts. Paper presented to 7th Annual National Nurse Managers Update Conference, Las Vegas, 31 March–2 April 1997.

RECOMMENDED READING

Campbell D (1982): Nursing the Aborigines. *Nursing Times* Dec.: 2019-2022

Carter E (1987): Borning: Pmere Laltyeke Ampe Mpwaretyeke — Congress Alukura by the Grandmother's Law. Canberra: Australian Aboriginal Studies.

Ellis J (1982): South East Asian refugees and maternity care — the Oakland experience. *Birth* 9 (3) Fall: 191-194.

Gilbert KR (1992): Religions as a resource for bereaved parents *Journal of Religion and Health* 31:19-30

Glover P (1986): Midwifery care in remote areas. *Australian Nursing Journal* 15 (10) May: 42-45.

Spector RE (1979): *Cultural Diversity in Health and Illness*. New York: Appelton-Century-Crofts.

INDEX